"Just as words cannot describe the [...] Universe" or "Divine Connection", to express how this book has touched [...] you and make sense of the fact that science and spirituality are connected in more ways than I imagined. This is a book to be shared with many, as long as I have a copy for my bedside table too." KEN CASLER

"It is sometimes the simplest things that crack me open when I realize them. Katrina's book Divine Union of the Masculine and Feminine is one such simple cracking-open. Gently paced and reflective, its chapters give the reader an opportunity to re-define and re-structure aspects of the Self no matter where they are on their life journey. This book is written for me and it's written for you, whoever you are!" AARTI ARIA MATHUR

"Katrina weaves from massive and diverse philosophies and paradigms but presents them into easy-to-understand and applicable offerings. Reading this book is like spending a delightful and heart-opening day with a wise and caring friend. I was able to immediately integrate the concepts in my life and challenge some of my unhelpful beliefs. By applying ideas on how the masculine can support the feminine, I have started to pave my way into self-mastery. If you feel stuck in any way, shape, or form, this book could be the answer!" MARY LLENELL PAZ ANORICO

"Absolutely brilliant! Katrina has captured and expressed the dance between the Divine union of the masculine and feminine in such a way that my soul was enraptured by the flow of love that carries the words. Indescribable, yet, I feel, a knowing, that resonates deep within my being. This book has kissed my soul, I'm feeling connected, inspired and ready to get out there and play. May this book be a spark of inspiration as it has been in my life." ALMA DIAZ

"In a world that keeps changing in such a fast pace, with new technologies emerging and making it possible for us to receive way more information than our brains can process, it is easy for us to feel compelled to do more, better, and faster, and to disconnect from our body, heart and soul in order to meet needs and expectations from others. Katrina's book is a kind invitation for us to slow down, reconnect with ourselves, and rethink and redefine the principles we have adopted to guide our lives that may no longer make sense. By learning more about Feminine and Masculine energies, how they operate within us, reflect in our relationships, and are expressed in the world, we can find our own ways to integrate them within us and open ourselves to infinite possibilities." KAREN EMY AOYAGUI

"Divine Union of the Masculine and Feminine" is a powerful, detailed look at the masculine and feminine dynamic in our society. Inclusive of all genders and orientations, Katrina Bos details how we have become unbalanced within ourselves, and gives us methods to rebalance our inner masculine and feminine in order to become whole - the key to finding inner bliss. From this blissful place within, we are able to shift into our natural polarity, whether masculine or feminine, and merge with another soul in divine union. Katrina takes us on a joyous intimate journey through the possibilities this polarizing can bring to our lovemaking and intimate relationships. Packed with stories from Katrina's personal journey, as well as introspective exercises for the reader to use to dig deep within themselves, this book is a fabulous guide for anyone looking to improve and deepen their personal and intimate relationships, and elevate them to a cosmic level. Highly recommended!" MELISA GLASSFORD

Divine Union of the Masculine & Feminine

By Katrina Bos

Divine Union of the Masculine & Feminine
Copyright ©2023 by Katrina Bos Productions Inc.

All rights reserved. No part of this publication may be reproduced, distributed, or transmitted in any form or by any means, including photocopying, recording, or other electronic or mechanical methods, without the prior written permission of the author, except in the case of brief quotations embodied in critical reviews and certain other non-commercial uses permitted by copyright law.

Cover Artist: Gina Maray

ISBN
978-1-7390401-0-9 (Paperback)
978-1-7390401-2-3 (Hardcover)
978-1-7390401-2-3 (eBook)

To all the wonderful people
who have let me share
in their hearts and lives.

Table of Contents

INTRODUCTION 1

SECTION I: CREATING A NEW FOUNDATION 7
- Chapter 1: Our Journey To Oneness 9
- Chapter 2: Redefining the Masculine & Feminine 21
- Chapter 3: Types of Loving Connection 33

SECTION II: THE MASCULINE & FEMININE DYNAMICS 45
- Chapter 4: Giving & Receiving 47
- Chapter 5: Talking & Listening 69
- Chapter 6: Structure & Chaos 85
- Chapter 7: Protector & Vulnerable 113
- Chapter 8: Leading & Following 131

SECTION III: FINDING BALANCE WITHIN 145
- Chapter 9: Inner Happiness 147
- Chapter 10: Doing & Being 153
- Chapter 11: Logic & Intuition 159
- Chapter 12: Inspiration & Manifestation 165

SECTION IV: SEXUAL INTIMACY & DIVINE UNION 173
- Chapter 13: Romantic Relationships 175
- Chapter 14: The Passion of Pursuit 183
- Chapter 15: Leading & Following In Intimacy 203
- Chapter 16: Giving & Receiving In Intimacy 211
- Chapter 17: Structure & Chaos In Intimacy 219

SECTION V: A DEEPER DIVE INTO THE MASCULINE & FEMININE 227
- Chapter 18: Archetypes of the Masculine & Feminine 229
- Chapter 19: Strengthening Our Masculine 235
- Chapter 20: Strengthening the Feminine 249
- Chapter 21: Removing the Domination Paradigm 261

SECTION VI: GOING ABOVE & BEYOND 267
- Chapter 22: An Intimate Connection with Our World 269
- Chapter 23: Becoming Something Brand New 277

About the Author 279
About the Cover Artist 281
Other Books by Katrina Bos 283

Introduction

> *"At the moment of orgasm*
> *The truth is illumined-*
> *The one everyone longs for.*
> *Lovemaking is riding the currents of excitation*
> *Into revelation.*
> *Two rivers flow together,*
> *The body becomes quivering.*
> *No inside and no outside -*
> *Only the delight of union.*
> *The mind releases itself into divine energy*
> *And the body knows where it came from.*
> *This is reality, and it is always here.*
> *Everyone craves the source,*
> *And it is always everywhere."*
> LORIN ROCHE, The Radiance Sutras

Can you imagine the excitement of what is happening in the quote above? "The truth is illumined... riding the currents of excitation... delight of union... the mind releases into divine energy... this is reality."

This is why I'm excited to share these teachings about the masculine and feminine. This and so much more is possible when these two beautiful polarities play and dance together!

The first time I heard this quote was at a tantra retreat in Big Sur, California. I was sitting with a couple hundred other people listening to Lorin Roche (the author) read these passages, first in Sanskrit and then in English. As I sat there, my whole body quivered in the way that tells you that you are hearing something very old and true. It is like the sensation of your hair standing on end when you hear a perfect piece of music. Your whole being aligns with something much greater and, going forward, you are a little bit different than you were a few moments before.

> *"No inside and no outside -*
> *Only the delight of union.*
> *The mind releases itself into divine energy*
> *And the body knows where it came from."*

Can you imagine feeling this total delight? The delight of inner union? The feeling of divine energy running through your body?

This might sound a bit "out there", but this is fully within our human experience. We are capable of amazing things — far beyond what we have been told or even imagined.

My Beginning

> *"Lovemaking is riding the currents of excitation*
> *Into revelation.*
> *Two rivers flow together,*
> *The body becomes quivering."*

There was a moment, decades before that day in California, when my soon-to-be husband and I were making love in my dorm room at University. We didn't seem to be doing anything different than normal but all of a sudden, our bodies merged together, disappeared, and we became the "two rivers flowing together" from the quote above. We felt bliss like we'd never felt before. It was beyond understanding. It almost seemed like we were in another dimension.

It would be 10 years later that I discovered tantra and started to understand what had happened that wonderful evening. Up until then, we had tried everything we could think of to replicate the experience, but to no avail. The problem was that we couldn't get there based on our current understanding of intimacy, relationships, being human, or anything about the world. It was like we were trying to build something on the wrong foundation.

Studying and practising tantra changed all that. The world around me became more expansive and incredible. More was possible in intimate relationships than we ever could have fathomed or read on the covers of magazines. My mind exploded as I tried to integrate the idea that we were divine, infinite beings into my day-to-day life, raising my children, working on the farm, and my marriage.

Most importantly, this is where I first heard about the masculine and feminine described in different ways than before. I had studied the yin and yang of Chinese philosophies and had certainly witnessed what society considered masculine and feminine (which are really just dysfunctional gender stereotypes), but now I was hearing about how the masculine and feminine dance together. I was learning about how they energize and serve each other, and how, if we can fully surrender to this dance, we will merge together and experience total bliss.

Although I was a long way from being able to replicate what they were talking about, my whole being knew that this was true. I knew that we were barely scratching the surface when it came to sexual intimacy, our connection to the Universe, and our own happiness.

Divine Union in Relationships

One of the big reasons we are drawn to study the Divine Union of the Masculine and Feminine is because we know that more is possible in romantic relationships. We have watched our parents, grandparents, neighbours, and friends have typical relationships for their generation. Maybe they initially married because they were in love, pregnant, or because that's just what people did. Then, over time, their relationship became like loving siblings, fighting siblings, distant, or just stagnant. On occasion, you might meet a couple who had been together for decades and who were actually happy and their relationship was dynamic and growing, but these are very few and far between.

And so, after witnessing this, we realize that we want more, but we're missing something. We know what we don't want, but that isn't enough to build something new. We need a different foundation than our ancestors.

The problem is that we don't know exactly what is missing.

We say that we want to make love and not just have sex, but what does that really mean? We want our partners to pursue us and make us feel loved, but then we are considered needy. We know that sexual intimacy should be incredible, dynamic, and make us feel closer than ever. Yet, it often becomes very robotic until it is non-existent.

This is where the magic of the true masculine and feminine comes in. When we understand how two beings are literally attracted to each other magnetically, we easily find the words to share with our partner so that we can explore new frontiers together. More importantly, by exploring the polarity that we prefer, we strengthen and expand the deepest parts of ourselves bringing us to a whole new level of confidence and joy in life.

Feeling Happiness Within

These masculine and feminine energies also exist within us. When they are beautifully balanced and dancing together, we feel the inner contentment and confidence that really allows us to live life to the fullest.

However, we have lived with a great separation within ourselves for centuries. In many religions, we are taught that we have a good side and a bad side. This belief can cause us to spend our lives with our "good" side suppressing our "bad" side. In many ways, this is also our inner masculine (taking on the role of the authority that taught this to us) oppressing our inner feminine (which holds our truth, emotions, dreams, and who we truly are).

INTRODUCTION

This sets up a great battle that wages within us for our whole life. Our inner masculine punishes our feminine (like we have experienced in the world). Our inner masculine judges our feminine causing us to not trust ourselves. Our inner masculine tries to control our wild and untamed side, cutting us off from freedom and our own mystery. Even the teaching that sexuality is wrong and thought to be a sin creates deep inner judgement, guilt, and cuts us off from so much love, pleasure, and personal power.

Instead, when our inner masculine and feminine are in union, our masculine protects our feminine allowing us to rest. Our masculine manifests the dreams and ideas of the feminine, allowing us to make our unique mark in the world. Our masculine trusts and loves our wild and mysterious side making life an ever-exciting adventure into the unknown.

This union within is actually the foundation of all of our peace and happiness. And luckily, this is also where we have the most power to make change.

Union with God, the Universe & Everything

All the dynamics in this book also allow us to connect with the amazing world around us. This is our ultimate communion. This is where we never feel alone. This is where we know that we belong because we feel it in every cell of our being.

This was a huge part of my journey in 1999, when I was sick and I met my first spiritual teacher, Jim. At this point, God, the Divine, etc. was really just an intellectual idea that made sense to me, but I had no actual connection, let alone union. Through my healing journey, I learned that there was actually deep wisdom within me that I could tap into. When I took action based on that wisdom, miracles began appearing in my life. It was so common that, when things lined up serendipitously, my husband, children, and friends would just laugh and say, "Yep, welcome to Katrina's world!"

I wrote the book *What If You Could Skip the Cancer?* in order to share my inner journey because people often asked me how I healed. They wanted to know the formula so that they, too, could heal. However, I didn't have any such formula. My journey had been from my head to my heart in order to access something much greater in the world. I had to shift how I saw the Universe, from the limited version that my brain could understand to trusting my feelings and hunches because that was where Divine wisdom lived.

Every time I listened within and took action, trusting that guidance got a little bit easier. I realized that I could trust this connection that was forming. Although I couldn't tell you what exactly I was connected to, with every experience the connection became deeper and almost visceral. All I knew was this: when I listened within, there was guidance there that I had never heard from anyone or read in a book. It was perfect for my situation every time and created healing with whoever was there.

I experienced Divine Union within. I still do today, and it changed my path completely.

When we connect with the Divine, Highest Self, Zen, Consciousness, or Spirit within, we realize that we are so much more than we ever thought. Life takes on an infinite dimension that becomes easier and easier to explore which makes life so exciting, expansive, and full of possibilities.

The feeling of this magical connection is the same when we connect with God, with someone we love, and within ourselves. This Divine Union is possible for all of us in all aspects of our lives.

So, we must create a new foundation to build upon. We must redefine the masculine and feminine, connection, and union.

From here, anything is possible!

SECTION I

Creating a New Foundation

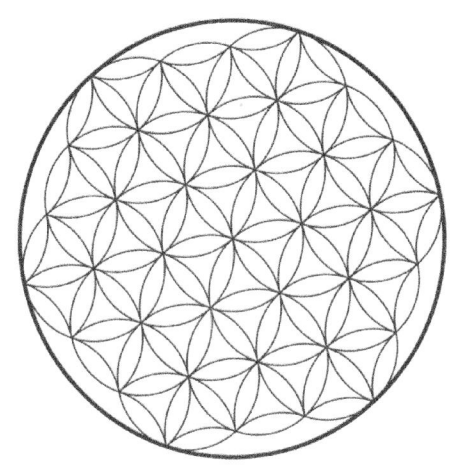

Chapter 1

Our Journey To Oneness

*The masculine and feminine
do not exist in isolation.
They play together
Building upon each other.
Most powerful when they polarize
Uniting in the bliss of oneness
And new creation.*
KATRINA BOS

We are meant for great connection.

We have lived in a paradigm of false separation for centuries. This causes the disconnect within us that makes us feel less than perfect. It disconnects us from the world around us, making us feel like we don't belong and feeling very alone in what we are going through. It also causes distance in our loving relationships, making us unable to connect deeply with those we love the most.

But none of this is real. Passion in relationships is meant to grow and deepen our connection. All that we are inside is meant to dance and play and build upon each other as we self-actualize, expand, and grow into who we truly are.

However, this is not the world that most of us have lived in. Although we know that we desire something more connected and joyful, we don't know how to create it within our lives. Therefore, we have to go back to first principles. We need to look at what we were taught by our families, society, churches, and schools. We need to look at the building blocks upon which everything we understand has been built.

We need to know that we are made for connection and true union. To make this happen, we must redefine the masculine and feminine, union, and what is truly possible within and between us all.

Connection, Union, & Divine Union

What is union? Is it simply being together or is it something more?

When we look at the classic yin-yang symbol, we see dualities such as light/darkness, hot/cold, and expansion/contraction. These dualities, held side by side, account for everything in the world. Everything is either light or dark, hot or cold, or somewhere on the continuum between the two.

A lot of our ideas about union are like this. As couples, we consider ourselves to be together because we are side by side. He takes care of the kids while I go to work. She likes to cook and I like to clean. I am extroverted and he is introverted. We work well together. These relationships follow the yin-yang complementary opposite pattern, and it makes for wonderful living, playing, and working together.

However, in this book, we are going to talk about a different kind of complementary opposites—masculine and feminine. These characteristics are all about magnetism, connection, and union.

Masculine and feminine are opposites in life, but are not part of a continuum. They are completely different. They attract, feed, nourish, and build each other and are attracted to each other like two poles of a magnet.

The strength of the magnetism can be of varying degrees. You might simply experience a gentle attraction with someone that turns into fun flirting at a party. Or maybe you have a stronger attraction to someone and it won't let you go. You pursue this person and create a friendship or loving relationship. Or, you may experience the ultimate divine union where, as you dance together, the magnetism becomes stronger and stronger, your energies become closer and closer until the line between you disappears completely, and you merge together into a greater oneness.

This is Divine Union.

This is the passion that two lovers feel as they begin to discover and trust each other. This is the joy of finding a leader whom we love to follow and, by doing so, we expand into greater versions of ourselves. This is the bliss of sitting with an old friend, talking over coffee as the hours disappear in loving friendship.

This is the nirvana that an artist feels as inspiration flows through them; they stand before their easel with paint and brushes, and their vision flows effortlessly onto the canvas. With every stroke, the inspiration grows even more. Soon, hours have gone by, and the artist sits back in pure euphoria, staring at the beautiful manifestation before them.

Divine union is walking outside in the springtime with the sunshine warming your face. As you take a deep breath in, you receive the sun's warmth, and then you exhale completely feeling totally in bliss.

This is sitting in meditation or prayer and surrendering ourselves completely to something greater. To open ourselves and to receive guidance. To know that we are part of something wonderful. To feel completely held by the Universe, God, and the quantum field.

Living in Duality

Current scientific theory says that we live in a space-time continuum. This allows each of us to be in different places on the Earth and experience life chronologically—or "over time". However, when pondering the true nature of time, many scientists wonder if time is even real as we know it or if all time is stacked on top of itself in a kind of cylinder, and everything is actually happening at once. Is the purpose of the space-time continuum to experience our lives in bite-size pieces even though it may be an illusion?

Similarly, spiritual teachers discuss the difference between being "in oneness" versus living "in duality". They say that "We are all One," and at the same time, we are each on individual paths.

When we live in Oneness, this is the "singularity." This is God-space, the quantum field, infinity, and the stillness that you feel within your heart. This is where God is omnipotent, omnipresent, and omniscient. This dimension of life is impossible to describe because our words are based in the physical world. This is why when we try to describe the singularity or anything transcendental, we tend to use poetry or other descriptive language to try to express the essence of what we've experienced. Our regular day-to-day language cannot do it justice.

If we imagine living in the singularity, we realize that we can't experience anything else because everything is One. And so, duality is created. The Oneness splits into the many, and now, we can all experience each other. Humans can experience other humans, animals, mountains, and chocolate.

This duality is our physical world. It allows us to experience ourselves over time. We were different yesterday than we are today. Duality is me writing this book and you reading it. It is being able to talk to my sister, do jigsaw puzzles with my children, and make love with my lover. Duality is all of our interactions with each other and the world around us.

Even though we are separate people in this duality, this connection to Oneness is also our nature. This is why the feeling of separation is our deepest wound. Somehow, we know that we are meant to be connected. We know that our interactions should bring us closer. We know that great joy and inner happiness could happen all the time, but we have seen this so seldom, we often wonder if it is possible at all.

The question becomes, *how do we experience it?* How can we experience the joy of Oneness within our day-to-day lives? Within our physical world? Within duality?

First, we must understand the driving force of the journey to union — magnetic attraction.

Magnetism

We are all made up of atoms which are essentially light energy — the singularity. Atoms are held close together by magnetic attraction. They are not even touching. They are just magnetically charged and heavily attracted to each other.

When I was a child and first learned about atomic theory, I pictured everyone as people made out of bubbles. Later, it blew my mind to realize that we weren't even bubbles. We were just the energy inside. I couldn't even fathom it! To think that our physical bodies, our ability to speak or to ride a bike was just energy held together by magnetism — that on some level there's no actual physical reality. How was that possible?

So, now let's imagine that this energy that makes up the atoms is the singularity (the Oneness). What we see around us is how the singularity expresses itself in this physical world.

Now, let's look closer at magnetism.

We know that there is a positive and negative pole to any magnet, and that the negative pole (feminine) draws the positive pole

CREATING A NEW FOUNDATION

(masculine) into it. These two opposite, yet attractive, polarities, are the foundation of all creation. When we explore our reality even deeper through quantum mechanics, we find out that no one actually understands how these charged particles act within the atom. They can disappear, appear in two places at once, and act in ways that make no sense at all. The mystery of what we are made of goes deeper and deeper the more we look into it.

However, in the physical world around us, we can observe many simple facts about magnetism. We know that positive and negative (masculine and feminine) are attracted to each other. We know that if you have two negatives, there is no magnetism and nothing happens. We also know that two positives repel each other.

You must have opposites to come together to create a bond. It is the same between us. This is why masculine and feminine energies attract each other.

We even use these magnetic terms in relationships. We say that we are attracted to that person but repulsed by another. We say that there is a real spark between us or that the spark has fizzled out. Unconsciously, we know that this magnetism is important in the excitement and potential of any relationship.

It is important to know that I am not talking about genders here or sexual orientation. We are talking about energy. If someone is very receptive (feminine) and someone else has something to share (masculine) then there is magnetic attraction. If two people are very receptive (feminine), nothing happens, and if two people are in their masculine, there is only battle. You need to have the difference for creation to happen. This is magnetism.

Masculine & Feminine In Separation

Somewhere in our history, most people stopped experiencing what it was to genuinely connect with another person. We knew how it was to live side by side. We knew how to get along well enough, but there was seldom any merging, bonding, or heart connection. There was no trust or deep love.

We ended up walking through life with our children, partners, and family like ships passing in the night. Even though we were doing things together—going on holidays, having sex, and eating meals—there was no actual connection. We had normalized this kind of co-living—that a bit (or a lot) of distance between us was totally normal.

When we look at the dynamics in this book, we have all experienced them in one way or another. We have been having conversations. We have been protected by people. We have been in relationships. We have been hurt and maybe even hurt others.

The reason we have been hurt—the reason relationships haven't always been joyful—is that we weren't actually connected. We were acting upon each other in total separation.

When we interact with people in separation, we are able to hurt them because we are not empathically feeling them. They are energetically "over there." They are just an object in our lives. They might even be our persecutor, dependant, or judge and jury. Although we might be married to them, everyone is just playing a role. There is no actual relating or relationship happening. And so, we can hurt each other and even tell ourselves that they deserve it.

But, as soon as we are in connection, we can't hurt each other because we can feel each other. This is why when we are in union, there is no need for guards, to be afraid, or worry. We can be wide open with each other. We know that the other person deeply gets us. What follows is just love, kindness, and ever-deepening connection.

Removing the Idea of Domination

Part of this separation is due to the domination paradigm we've been living within. Not only are we separate from others, but we try to dominate them. This is something that we have lived with for generations and so it is often hard to tease out of our personalities. But we have to unearth it within ourselves as we explore these

CREATING A NEW FOUNDATION

dynamics because if we are unconsciously afraid that we will be dominated, we will not want to be on the feminine side of any of the dynamics, and if we are afraid to be seen as the dominating partner, we will shy away from the masculine polarity.

This can lead us to being afraid of being in either the masculine or feminine polarity, and then we are left with nothing. No charge. No excitement. We experience stagnation in life, both internally and in our relationships.

This is why it is important to look at where this comes from so that we can remove the pattern from our internal programming and all of our relationships.

It's hard to say when this desire to dominate began. We have had empires around the world for thousands of years. There are a few stories of benevolent rulers, but most were more of the dominating character. Many countries have royal families who are held above the "regular class." There is an "elite" class of people who control the money in the world which creates a paradigm of "haves" and "have-nots."

In many of our world's governments, the desire for domination creates a huge separation between the masculine and feminine. Ideally, the government (masculine) is there to take care of the people (feminine). However, the government dynamic is more like the master-servant—or "tyrant king" relationship. In this polarity flip, the people serve the king. The people are taxed to serve those in power, and if they don't pay, the military is brought in to make sure they do. We can see this flipped "tyrant" dynamic not only in government but in families where the man is the head of the household or a boss in a business. The one "in charge" creates the rules and those "beneath" must follow them or else.

All of these systems create the foundation of a power struggle. Nobody wants to be the one without power. Nobody wants to have to serve another without choice.

This domination idea has crept into our definition of the masculine and feminine as well. There is the idea that the masculine is dominant and the feminine is submissive, that the masculine has the power and the feminine has none.

But this isn't true.

Both polarities are powerful. Masculine energy has power. Feminine energy has power. All genders have power. All people are inherently powerful to create their lives. This is absolutely necessary to understand if we want to experience union with others. Otherwise, we will either impose our desire to dominate or our fear of powerlessness upon all of the energy dynamics that we're learning.

For example, when we look at the dynamic of leading and following, if we see this through the lens of a power struggle, the leaders have power, and the followers have none. But this isn't true. Each simply has a different role to play in the dance. Both are equally powerful.

In the protector-vulnerable dynamic, each is equally powerful. In nature, the male lion protects the lioness when she has cubs with her. On her own, she is very powerful. But after she has given birth and must protect her offspring, the male lion will focus on fending off attacks. His dedication to her and her trust in his strength creates a union that protects the next generation of cubs. Both parents are equally powerful. Her job is to care for the cubs. His job is to keep predators away.

We can see this in human situations too. There are times in our lives when we are struggling because we have too much on our plates. We need help. There is too much for one person to do. This is a great opportunity to ask for help. This is the feminine asking the masculine for what is needed—maybe time, food, skills, or financial help.

This giving and receiving can be a beautiful union, but neither role is more powerful than the other. One simply has a need and the other has what is needed—a beautiful opportunity for meaningful connection.

Happiness Comes from Union, Not Power

Joy and happiness do not come from power.

We often believe that power will bring us happiness because that's what we have been taught by a world that only values power and control. We spend our lives seeking more and more no matter how much we already have. Sometimes we seek power for the thrill or security we believe it brings, but often we just don't want to be controlled by others.

The bottom line is that we each must have the autonomy to live according to our soul's purpose. Our freedoms are often overtly and subtly stripped from us by those in authority, and so, on a soul level, we know that we must fight for this autonomy.

But in the end, this quest for power doesn't bring us to bliss. It might spare us the suffering of oppression, but it doesn't allow us to actually grow in life. When we seek power or fear another's control, we end up unable to connect deeply with them or anyone else. When we are forever wanting to have the upper hand, we seldom take the time to look within and begin the journey to true inner happiness.

Instead, let's imagine that we are whole and fully balanced within. We aren't seeking power, we don't fear others, and we would love to authentically engage with other people. Maybe you see a need in your community to have a centre where the kids could gather. What is the next step? You could go home and start sketching out the ideal community centre on your own. Or, you could call together the kids who inspired you in the first place and ask them what *they* would love to have in a community centre.

When we see a need and then connect with those we want to help, this is our masculine reading the feminine. Yes, you could just draw up the plans in private, build the community centre, and sit back and be content that you did a good thing. Instead, when you connect with the folks who will be using it, you create much more than a community centre. You create connections with others. The kids feel your respect for their ideas. The parents know that you are listening to them too. This respect inspires you as well, and this beautiful positive feedback loop expands upon itself, nourishing and bonding with everyone involved.

It is this bliss within the connection that brings us true happiness.

Similarly, imagine you are a teacher. You could simply present your teachings to the class regardless of who is there. Or you could begin the class by asking the students to each share a bit about themselves and maybe what they would like to learn about the subject? You would start to get a feel for the mix of everyone present. You would start to hear the real questions in the room. From here, you can still share what you intended to teach, but you will do it differently. You will include stories that specifically address the questions asked. You will teach it in a different spirit than you would have had you stayed "in separation."

For example, imagine you are giving a lecture about the effects of sexual abuse on teenagers. To be truly helpful, you must know who is in your audience. What would you share if you were teaching a room full of psychologists who were working with abused teens? What if the room was filled with abused teenagers or their parents? What if you were talking to a group of abusers in prison? Or what if you were speaking to twelve-year-old kids who could potentially be future victims?

To connect with your audience (the feminine), you (the masculine) will tailor your teachings to the group. From here, you can share help and true wisdom. The audience will know that you are talking directly to them, and they will ask deeper questions. The whole experience is transformed from something that could have been very dry and unimportant to something incredibly meaningful and impactful on people's lives.

This is the joy of connection and union.

CREATING A NEW FOUNDATION

Your Personal Journey:

Please use these questions as prompts for personal journaling, discussions with friends or partners, or group study.

1. Have you felt disconnection within yourself? Like your "good" side and "bad" side are distanced and conflicted? What would union feel like within yourself?
2. Have you felt separation in relationships? With romantic partners, family, parents, or children? Where do you desire union with others the most?
3. How would your life change if you embraced the idea that there was no such thing as time? What would living in that Oneness feel like?
4. Have you experienced magnetism with other people? Who have you been magnetically attracted to? Who have you been repulsed by?
5. Have you experienced this domination paradigm in your life? Was it like this within your family growing up? In romantic relationships? At work? In school or church?
6. Have you ever experienced true union with someone else — where you are both totally connected and there is only joy? Who was it?
7. Do you feel comfortable with the idea of deep connection with others?

CHAPTER 2

REDEFINING THE MASCULINE & FEMININE

"Know the masculine. Keep to the feminine."
LAO TZU

The above quote is very important for our study. Within this separation paradigm, the feminine was often oppressed or denied. This has appeared as the oppression of women, children, employees, slaves, servants, and vulnerable members of any society. We see this in ideas, too. We see logic (masculine) as being more important than intuition (feminine), what we know (masculine) being preferred over mystery (feminine), or structure (masculine) being preferred over chaos (feminine).

We will see this pattern throughout all of the dynamics in this book. In many places in our lives, we can see this repression (and sometimes even fear) of the feminine, which not only creates painful separation between each other, but also causes us to ignore who we are at our core.

As we redefine the masculine, we will look at how this energy acts in connection with the feminine. Most of the masculine energy we have known in our lives has been in this separation that causes pain, oppression, and division. This is why many of us shy away from being in the masculine role—we have seen it at its worst, and we aren't sure how to embrace it in a healthy way.

As we discuss the feminine, we must redefine it as well (or define it as it always should have been) because we may only understand it as it pertains to the unhealthy, detached masculine. And so, in the same way that we may avoid being in the masculine role, we may avoid being in the feminine as well.

Masculine & Feminine Are About Connection

In the past, we may have thought that masculine and feminine had something to do with traits of genders. Masculine was burly, strong, aggressive, angry, and could even include violent "manly" behaviour. The feminine was anything that the manly types desired—curvy, weak, quiet, submissive, demure, and emotional.

These are not masculine and feminine. These are just aspects of the domination culture that we have had to play a part in through gender.

Masculine and feminine are simply two sides of any human connection. These two energies are magnetically attracted to each other in healthy, serving ways, and, depending on the situation, can create total bliss when we openly surrender to them.

Let's take an example from the giving-receiving dynamic. Imagine you are visiting a friend's place and your stomach starts to growl. Your friend says, "Hey, are you hungry?" You reply, "Yes, actually." Your friend then offers to make you a sandwich. She gives you the sandwich and your hunger is satisfied. In this dynamic, she is the masculine giver and you are the feminine receiver. A warm and fuzzy connection is made because masculine energy satisfied a feminine need in the world.

Let's imagine a similar scenario but within the domination paradigm. You are sitting with someone when they get up to make a salami sandwich. They then return and give it to you to eat. You respond that you aren't hungry or that you don't like salami. The person in the masculine (the giver) says, "But I made you a sandwich! You should eat it! You're too skinny. You need to eat!" And you say, "But I'm not hungry."

You can see the disconnection between the two people. The giver simply wants to impose what they have upon the other. This same disconnected "giving" pattern shows up when we give unsolicited advice, when we want to have sex when our partner isn't interested, or when someone won't stop talking and we feel obligated to listen.

If we have had a lot of this disconnected, forced giving, we may choose total independence from others. If someone offers us a metaphorical sandwich, we will simply say no. We don't want the strings attached. We don't want other people messing in our lives. It is easier to just withdraw and disconnect completely from the world.

The key is that in a connected space, the masculine and feminine satisfy each other. The masculine has something to give, and the feminine desires something. They are completely complementary, and together, they create a happier situation than before. There is no power struggle or worry of domination because neither person is always in the masculine or the feminine. At any time, either person may be in either role. It all depends on the situation.

Masculine & Feminine Are Not About Gender

Using these words can be problematic because we generally think of masculine being about men and feminine being about women. There are a few situations where gender might play a role in heterosexual relationships, but in most cases, gender is irrelevant.

We could also use the terms yin and yang or positive and negative, but neither of these pairings is quite right either.

CREATING A NEW FOUNDATION

Yin and yang are the most common descriptions of the masculine and feminine and come out of the Taoist tradition. They represent how the opposites in life must always be in balance. As we can see in the chart, some of these pairs are simply the opposite of the other and others have some flow from one to the other. But these don't describe the dynamic relationship that we are looking for that brings us into union.

Yin	Yang
dark	light
cool	hot
passive	active
night	day
moon	sun
descending	rising
form	energy
interior	exterior

The terms positive and negative refer to the two poles of a battery. These are closer to what we want because they describe actual magnetism. The positive pole is attracted to the negative pole in a very real and tangible way. Plus, this relationship describes how some things attract or repulse each other. However, due to our common use of "positive" meaning good and "negative" meaning bad, I imagine that we would run into even more challenges than we do with the words masculine and feminine.

As we go forward, we will redefine the masculine and feminine as complementary opposites with a magnetic charge that dance together, closer and closer with the possibility of creating total union.

Here are the dynamics that we will be discussing in this book:

Masculine	Feminine
giving	receiving
talking	listening
structure	chaos
protector	vulnerable
leading	following
pursuer	pursued
manifestation	inspiration
logic	intuition
doing	being
Divine	human

There is an activity and magnetism that connects these pairs. They are not two sides of the same coin. They are complementary like two ends of a magnet which create a polarity that draws each to the other until they merge completely.

Most of the time, the situation will determine whether we are in the masculine or the feminine role. Sometimes we are the giver and other times, we receive. Sometimes, we are the vulnerable one, and other times, we are the strong shoulder to cry on. Most of the time, we easily fluctuate between both poles.

However, in romantic relationships, there will be one partner who prefers and is strengthened by being in the masculine polarity and the other who prefers to explore the feminine. In heterosexual relationships, it is most often the man who is strengthened by exploring the masculine polarity and the woman who is strengthened in the feminine. In same-sex couples, there will be one partner who prefers the masculine and the other who prefers the feminine.

However, it is important to note that this preference is only for the romantic part of their relationship. It has nothing to do with household chores, caring for children, or who makes the decisions in the relationship. For couples where romance isn't desired, this preference doesn't apply. They will just flow back and forth in the dynamics depending on the situation.

We will go deeper into this preference discussion later.

Pink Jobs & Blue Jobs

A man once told me that he was confused about his polarity preference because he believed that he wanted to be in the masculine. Yet he always found himself in the "nurturing feminine" role in relationships.

But nurturing is not a feminine role. Nurturing is the masculine energy of caring for someone else even though it is often done by women.

We have often considered the things that our moms did to be feminine and what our dads did to be masculine. According to this, "pink jobs" like caring for children and cooking are feminine jobs and "blue jobs" like building fences and taking out the garbage are masculine jobs.

However, all of these are masculine. Doing, giving, and manifesting are all masculine. These tasks have nothing to do with polarity, preference, or gender. Splitting up the household chores is simply sharing the responsibilities of a household. Any group of people would do this regardless of gender in order to live together harmoniously.

These jobs were often split between genders in many societies, so we tend to get caught in the idea that certain jobs like nursing or secretarial work are feminine and being a doctor or driving a truck is masculine. However, these are just social constructs as to what each gender should be doing. All genders can do all of these jobs.

REDEFINING THE MASCULINE & FEMININE

They have nothing to do with the masculine and feminine that we are talking about.

It is interesting to note that there are times when certain jobs do line up better with one gender than another. In 1993, I married a dairy farmer. I was a 23-year-old computer programmer from Toronto and very comfortable as a woman "working in a man's world." I thought that splitting jobs based on gender was ridiculous and I argued endlessly with anyone who thought differently. So, of course, I learned how to drive tractors, milk the cows, and do anything else that was considered "men's work," mostly on principle.

A few years later, I found myself with a baby on my back and a small child underfoot. I soon realized that when my children were nursing and then toddlers, it was better for them to be in the house—clean, safe, and with me. It made sense that my husband was out in the barn working with the livestock and big machinery without little ones around. It was seldom a safe place for children.

The division of labour on the farm based on gender made practical sense because I was the one breastfeeding and physically recovering from giving birth. There were definitely situations in our history (and today) where this makes sense.

However, as a rule, this division of labour continued in our lives long after we left the farms and there weren't any children underfoot. Housework became "women's work." Machinery, fixing the lawnmower, and climbing on the roof became men's work.

The feminist movement has done a lot to bring us out of these stereotypes realizing that men can change diapers and women can change the oil in the car. However, we need to stay aware that we still may have some of these stereotypes whispering in our ears from generations past.

The Masculine & Feminine Do Not Exist Separately

It is also important to know that the masculine and feminine are two parts of a whole. They do not exist separately.

We have often heard, "That person is very feminine or effeminate," or "That person is very masculine or manly." However, effeminate and manly are not the same as feminine and masculine. These words simply describe gender stereotypes and have nothing to do with energy, connection, or the dance of the masculine and feminine.

"Manly" tends to describe the patriarchal version of an ideal man — warrior build, stoic in temperament, and perhaps even prone to anger, aggression, and controlling behaviour — essentially, qualities of the patriarchy. Anything that is not like that is considered "effeminate", unmanly, oversensitive, soft, needy, and requiring someone (a man) to care for them.

It is interesting to note that the word effeminate has nothing to do with the feminine at all. In the Merriam-Webster dictionary, effeminate means "1. Having feminine qualities untypical of a man: not manly in appearance or manner, 2: marked by an unbecoming delicacy or overrefinement. I.e. Effeminate art, an effeminate civilization."

These definitions have nothing to do with connection, magnetism, or union. Unfortunately, they also give us no understanding of what feminine is. They only tell us that it isn't masculine, which disempowers the feminine aspect completely. Because of this, a large part of our study will be to understand the power and qualities of the feminine in our interactions and within all of us.

Masculine is Born of the Feminine

A foundational idea we have about the masculine and feminine is that the masculine is in charge, "driving the boat," so to speak, and that the feminine simply follows along. But understanding that the masculine is born from the feminine turns these old ideas upside down.

If the goal of our interaction is true connection and union, the masculine will choose what they do based on what the feminine needs, desires, intuits, etc. We feed someone (masculine) because they are hungry (feminine). We speak (masculine) because another person desires to hear something (feminine). We help (masculine) because someone needs help (feminine).

This is how we begin to experience the union of the masculine and feminine.

However, if the masculine simply imposes their desires upon the feminine, the feminine will naturally put up guards against anything unwanted. Everyone will be in separation. This is where we give advice that isn't asked for. This is where we interfere where we are not welcome. This is where we control or protect where it isn't needed or desired. In these situations, the feminine is just an object of their desire—sexually, career-wise, ego-wise, or in the pursuit of power.

This domination paradigm often shows up sexually. For centuries, in many Western societies, it was believed that women had no sex drives, nor were they capable of experiencing pleasure in sexual intercourse. So, of course, the men had to initiate, and the women had to comply whether they wanted to or not. It was their obligation through marriage. This, combined with the lack of birth control and programming from many churches saying that sex was sinful, left many women frigid and not wanting sex at all.

Imagine the difference today as we embrace our sexual wholeness and the masculine sees their feminine partner as a wealth of potential wisdom, intuition, and sensual pleasures. Sexual intimacy becomes an adventure of discovering their partner and themselves. Imagine the feminine partner knowing that they are fully in the game—that their current mood, desires, and reality are all important parts of the experience.

Just imagine what is possible there.

Being Both Masculine & Feminine

For some people, it is a lifelong goal to be considered either masculine or feminine. Perhaps we were raised by our parents to always be strong and in charge. Or maybe we were taught that always being soft and the peacekeeper was the ideal way to be. This is where we have to be very careful.

In romantic relationships, we have polarities that we prefer and have great joy in fully polarizing as we connect, dance, and merge with our lover. However, this polarization only exists within this merging. We don't want to get stuck there.

If we desire happiness within and true connection with others, our goal must be wholeness within ourselves, which means being fully balanced in our own masculine and feminine. It isn't until we come into contact with someone else that we shift into one polarity or the other.

We get into trouble when we define ourselves based on the polarity we prefer. Someone might walk around trying to "be masculine" whether they are interacting with anyone or not. Another person may want to be "always in the feminine." Both of these ways of moving through the world are out of balance.

Often, these people are simply playing into the stereotypes where the masculine is big and strong and the feminine is always sensual and demure. Or maybe they are utilizing the true masculine and feminine definitions that we are studying and the one wanting to be perceived as masculine must always be the protector, giver, and planner. While another, perpetually desiring to be in the feminine, always wants to receive, be in a vulnerable state, and have everything laid out for them.

One problem is, that by doing this, they are asking the world to always be in the opposite polarity regardless of the situation. The "ever-masculine" person needs everyone to need their protection, and the "ever-feminine" person will expect everyone to be doing things for them no matter what. Everyone in their lives is just an object playing a role in their ego's need to always be masculine or feminine.

However, the greater challenge is that they won't learn how to be in the opposite polarity. They will forever live a half-life—never experiencing their true potential. The "ever-masculine" person will never allow themselves to receive help, show emotions, or to be wild and untethered. Similarly, the "ever-feminine" person will never take charge, create structure in their lives, or seek logical solutions. They will want to be forever flowing "in their feminine".

These scenarios result in a personal imbalance. Yes, they will struggle in relationships and the workplace. But most importantly, they won't embrace both polarities within themselves, leaving them unbalanced from the inside out—forever seeking others to "make them feel complete".

Instead, we want to be fully balanced masculine and feminine within so that we can be whole, happy, and blissful all on our own. Then, as we go out into the world and interact with others, we can easily be in the masculine or the feminine role depending on the situation. We are flexible and able to respond to what's needed in the moment.

Your Personal Journey:

1. Are you easily connected with your feminine side? Your ability to receive? Be vulnerable? Be wild and full of mystery?
2. Are you easily connected with your masculine side? Always giving to others? Loving to manifest in the world? Do you enjoy logic and structure?
3. Do you tend toward one side or the other in life? Or are you pretty balanced?
4. What about in relationships? Do you prefer to be in the masculine or the feminine most of the time?

Chapter 3

Types of Loving Connection

*"When you make love, if you're lucky,
you'll have no idea whose body is whose.
And then both bodies will completely disappear
in the total bliss of lovemaking."*
~ JIM, *my first spiritual teacher*

What is Divine Union?

This is a kind of energetic union that combines two physical beings, and when lined up just right, you experience total bliss and ecstasy. There are many couples who have loving and kind connections (which is an awesome love to have), but here, we are talking about circulating energy as one.

The closest thing we can equate this to could be the moment of orgasm when you seem to leave this reality for a moment or two. You experience bliss or as the French would say "un petit mort" – a little death. The difference is that here, we are experiencing it with another person. It isn't a simultaneous orgasm. Instead, two people are experiencing the same orgasmic state together.

The key is to feel that magnetic attraction of true polarization, allow ourselves to be drawn to another, and then trust what might happen.

CREATING A NEW FOUNDATION

It's important to note that this polarization is different from what we might think. Sometimes, we use the term "polarization" to describe when people have opposing ideas about a discussion or an issue. There is the sense of repelling each other. This makes sense when we are living in separation from each other. Polarization, in that case, simply moves us further apart.

However, when people are connected and there is love and respect, then having a discussion where they hold opposite views becomes exciting and a learning opportunity. The conversation becomes a fascinating debate of ideas. Each person gains new understanding of the other, thus gaining more understanding of themselves. In fact, it often creates a much more interesting discussion than if both hold the exact same perspective.

The key is that each person doesn't have to change their mind and join the other because there is respect of the different perspectives.

This idea of polarization in connection will be a repeated theme for the rest of this book. Now let's imagine this in intimacy, where the polarity is between the masculine and feminine — two polarities that are naturally attracted together.

Devon and Jackie are sitting in front of each other. Each has their own individual energy that is nourishing and flowing through them in total balance. They are each their own complete yin/yang symbol — equally masculine and feminine. As they gaze into each other's eyes, they sense a magnetic attraction between them. There is a tug between their hearts to be closer to the other. There is a desire to touch and connect deeper. There is a quiet desire to merge.

Devon initiates movement. This masculine energy reaches out to caress the other. Jackie receives this touch in feminine receptivity and feels love. Relaxing into this touch, part of Jackie's masculine protectiveness releases. Devon feels this release and begins to stroke Jackie's hair.

With every masculine action, the feminine surrenders a little more. Their yin-yang symbols are starting to merge. Devon is giving up their yin energy and Jackie is giving up their yang.

At the beginning of this polarization, it feels wonderful. Each person enjoys what is being given and received. The touch and attention are exciting and they start to feel a nice flow between them. However, the more they polarize, the more challenging it can become. We are accustomed to being balanced within. It takes great trust in the other, ourselves, and the Universe to surrender this balance to merge with another person. So, as the polarization continues, we need deeper and deeper trust.

Bit by bit, layer by layer, we surrender to each other. The energy builds to an incredible crescendo of faith, fear, trust, and desire… and then you cross the threshold. Both people are fully polarized, and the world disappears around you. You are flying in infinity. There is white light and love all around. Your bodies no longer exist, and you fly together in total bliss.

This is divine union.

Types of Loving Connection

There are many kinds of relationships and they all serve different purposes. Some are disconnected to the point of being combative and cruel. Some are loving but they feel more like a kind of sibling, neutral energy. Others are passionate and full of eros. Others desire and are capable of divine union.

Relationships are a function of how balanced each person is within themselves. If we are unbalanced within, we will seek a co-dependent relationship in order to feel whole. If we have unresolved personal issues, we will easily end up in combative relationships to create the arena to work them out. However, if both people are fully balanced within and do not need to have a relationship to feel whole, then they are free to polarize and explore many interesting possibilities as a couple.

Let's look at how these different kinds of relationships work (or don't work) with Divine Union.

Disconnected Relationships

Many of our relationships in life are disconnected. There are walls up. There is sarcasm and "jokes with a jab." We can't share our true selves for fear of mockery or having that vulnerability used against us. There is no feeling of safety at all.

These could be our family of origin, friendships, colleagues, and romantic relationships.

The dynamics in this book don't apply within these disconnected relationships. Due to the inherent power struggles and desire for domination, all interactions in these relationships will come out with a twist. Giving and receiving will turn into forcing and submission. Protector and vulnerable will turn into control and impotence. Structure and chaos will turn into domination and mayhem.

Masculine and feminine dynamics assume a primary desire for true, loving connection. So, this is what first must be healed in any relationship. We must learn how to be kind. We must redefine love. We must redefine what is possible in relationships. I cover these topics at length in my book *Tantric Intimacy: Discover the Magic of True Connection*.

We will touch on the effects of these disconnections in later chapters, but in relationships where the masculine and feminine flourish, love must be there. Kindness must be there. Respect must be there. Equality must be there, or else no true connection or dance is possible, let alone merging or union.

So, let's look at the relationships where connection exists and the dance of the masculine and feminine is possible.

Loving Coexistence

This is a loving and joyful coexistence which is wonderful to experience. You care about each other. You are kind. You consider each other's needs and desires. You truly love each other and enjoy all of your interactions.

TYPES OF LOVING CONNECTION

All of the dynamics in this book happen effortlessly between you. People in joyful relationships naturally flow in all masculine and feminine dynamics. If someone is hurting, you are there for them. If you need something, the other provides it. No one is keeping score or forcing themselves on anyone. One person will play masculine structure for another person's feminine flow. One person's chaos will inspire another person's order.

This could be friendships, family members, and romantic partners. There is love, respect, and kindness. You are confidantes for each other and have each other's backs.

These relationships may be enjoyed simply as they are… or there might be more desired.

ROMANTIC LOVE: EROS

Eros is the beginning of the focused dynamic of the masculine and feminine. Just like you live, raise children, and go to family events together, eros is another aspect of your relationship. Oftentimes, in the busyness of life, eros can take a back seat, and sometimes it completely disappears. This is where "the spark goes out," even though there is love and kindness in the relationship.

Eros is the magnetism that draws us together. This requires the polarity of two magnets: positive and negative, masculine and feminine. This manifests in exciting romance. This is where the honeymoon never ends because magnetism keeps new things happening. The masculine pursues the feminine and the feminine is gloriously mysterious and loves receiving from the masculine.

Not all couples desire this kind of magnetic excitement. Many are completely happy with the previous kind of love, which is wonderful and quite an accomplishment in today's world.

In erotic magnetism, one partner will have a preference for the masculine and the other for the feminine. Attraction deepens (even after many years). On a day-to-day basis, little things continue to strengthen the connection and expand each person.

This does not apply to our whole life together—only the erotic aspects. In the rest of our lives, we flow between the masculine and feminine depending on what the situation warrants. Most of the time, each person is their whole self, interacting with the world. But when eros is online, passion excites and thrills!

Divine Union

Then there is divine union. Sometimes, within the erotic aspect of your lives, you have a chance to completely focus on each other. Within this bubble, the masculine can focus completely on giving and the feminine can focus on opening to receive. The masculine digs deep within to become the structure needed as the feminine surrenders to explore total chaos.

The closer we get to 100% polarization, the less we control, and the less we can describe until—poof—something happens: total union. There are no more bodies. The connection is there but neither of you exists any longer.

This may seem like something that doesn't happen very often, which is true, depending on your lifestyle and how often you get to play in this kind of intimate bubble.

But it is important to know that this is at one end of the continuum of what's possible in intimacy. It is the hope and spirit that lives within every bouquet of flowers, massage, and kind gesture. It is in every smile and blissful spooning. It is within the text message that promises an evening of romance.

It is part of our human potential and experience… if we desire it.

I and Thou—Seeing the Other as Whole

For us to have a true connection, we must consider each other as the complete and amazing humans that we are. This may seem obvious, but due to the separation we have been living in, we tend to treat each other as objects, as opposed to actual sentient beings. And sometimes, we don't even treat ourselves as whole humans—

objectifying ourselves—assuming that we are not worth being part of the equation.

Martin Buber wrote a book called *I and Thou* where he looks at how we relate to each other. He considers the following kinds of relationships: "I-Thou," "I-It," "It-It," and "It-Thou."

In theory, when we encounter an object, we would have an "I-It" experience. We are the "I" and the object is the "It." When we encounter a person, ideally, we would have an "I-Thou" relationship where we are the "I" and we consider the other a whole human worthy of deep respect—a "Thou." However, this is not always so. Some doctors, to keep some distance from their patients, may keep things at an "I-It" experience. On the other side, some people treat objects (like fancy cars) with an "I-Thou" reverence.

The key to interacting with anyone—children, lovers, parents, friends—is to have an "I-Thou" relationship. Buber says that we only *experience* an "It." We *react* to "It." We fight back or agree with "It." We might try to form or manipulate "It." But these are not genuine relationships. Alternatively, he says that we *relate* to a "Thou." We bring our whole selves into the picture. We consider this person with respect and honour. To relate to someone is to identify with and connect with them.

As a baby, we begin life in the unity of I-Thou. Then, as time goes on, we often experience many "I-It" relationships, which can be quite painful and this begins our feelings of disconnection in the world.

THE "I-IT" RELATIONSHIP

When we experience an "I-It" relationship, others are mere objects in our life—players on our chessboard. As on object, if you are my partner, you are simply a part of my life. I require you to fulfill a certain role for me because you are there for a specific purpose.

Often, the objectified person has to act a certain way, look a certain way, or have a certain kind of job. Sometimes, all that is needed is

CREATING A NEW FOUNDATION

that they are there, holding space, so that the other doesn't have to be alone.

Sometimes, this is how we treat children. We think that the children are a reflection of us. The child has to get the right education and the right job, marry the right person, and have a certain number of children. How our children look to the neighbours is more important than connecting and truly relating with what they are going through on the inside.

In schools, the teacher-student relationship is a clear masculine-feminine dynamic. The teacher is speaking, and the students are listening, absorbing what is being taught. Although there have always been teachers who are connected to the humanness of their students, on the whole, our education system treats the students as objects to be processed. The teachers must simply "get through the curriculum," and the children are then graded on how well they received and were able to repeat the information. The child is not considered a whole being who is there to learn. They are objects to be processed. This is why schools like Waldorf have been created so that children in their wholeness are considered. Their learning is tailored to them. They are not objects. They are complete humans.

How often are employees treated like objects who can be treated however management sees fit? In this case, they are playing out the "Leader-Follower" dynamic, but with no connection. The employees are just objects.

In many governments, the people of the country are simply a tax base and not individuals with hopes and dreams.

In parenting, there are always lovely exceptions, but for centuries, children were also treated as objects. Parents were put in the role of authority over them—to keep them in line. They were there for punishment and control. The children were considered "mouths to feed," and often, they were there to work on the farm. Even now, with many well-intentioned parents, what matters are the marks that the children get at school, which university they attend, or whether they play hockey or soccer.

Do these parents love their children? Sure, but we have often been trained to process our children into something that we can feel good about. There is a reason that so many cultures find the teen years so difficult as a parent. The teens will no longer accept being treated as objects to be moulded into whatever vision their parents have for them. They want to be seen for who they truly are. Unconsciously, they know that they have been cheated out of a real, connected relationship and instead have been treated as objects. Now they are adults and will not tolerate it.

This "I-It" experience is obvious when it shows up in our romantic relationships. How often is the other person treated like an object instead of a whole person? They are the breadwinner, or the trophy wife (or husband). They owe you sex and intimacy. We have expectations of each other. We have needs that we want the other to fulfill.

The "I-Thou" Relationship

"When we encounter another individual truly as a person, not as an object for use, we become fully human."
MARTIN BUBER

When we move to the "I-Thou" relationship, we are now relating to this other person. We are seeing this other person as a human being who is on a path. We are aware that they have desires, hopes, and dreams. They are not just a player in our world. They are a human being experiencing life on this planet. In this case, we relate to each other, as opposed to needing each other to be a certain way in our lives.

This was important when I began teaching Tantra. Many of the couples who struggled with achieving the deeper intimacy they were seeking, often had an "I-It" relationship. That is how they had sex, talked, went on holidays, and raised the kids together. The other person simply fulfilled something for the other. It wasn't evil. It's just all they had ever known.

CREATING A NEW FOUNDATION

However, the tantric perspective asks us to see the divine in each other. It asks us to slow down, look into each other's eyes, and see the human that is in front of us— to see the divine being that is naked with us. Now what will we do?

As I would chat with the couples, the women would tell me that they were unhappy because their husbands expected them to just show up, be horny, and have sex with them. There wasn't any dinner or foreplay or loving moments ahead of time. It was just simply, "Hey, we're in bed, do you wanna…?" Sex was an obligation they had to fulfill, and due to a lack of passion and magnetism, the women hadn't been attracted to their husbands for many years. So, they actually didn't want any sexual intimacy at all.

I would ask them why they stayed. Whether they had been together for five, ten, or thirty years, their response would be something like, "Well, I like the home we have, and I don't want to be single. I don't know what I would do alone." I started to realize that the "I-It" relationship was going the other way, as well. These men were providing a secure home and a comfortable lifestyle. And even if the women had money of their own, simply having their husbands in their lives kept them out of the single scene. So, this wasn't quite so victim-oriented or one-sided as I had thought.

It is important to note that these are all good people. The problem is that we have normalized these kinds of relationships. We have normalized that as long as our partner plays a nice enough role in our life, we can hang out with the grandchildren together, and we're pretty comfortable, then it's all good.

Yet both people have stopped trying to connect as humans—or maybe they never did. We have also normalized marrying someone because they "check all the right boxes." Maybe they have a good job, come from a good family, have similar goals, would never be unfaithful, and we are attracted to them sexually. Perhaps we don't want to be alone, we want to have children, or we want to have a home. Then someone comes along, they are good enough, the timing is right, and they "check enough boxes."

But is it the human that you love? Is it their spirit? Is it that soul that you want to connect with? If it's not, that's fine. If we are truly looking for an "I-It" relationship, that's cool. It's not about judgment. But, in an "I-It" relationship, we will never get to blend and experience deeper intimacy with each other. There will always be a limit.

Whereas, in an "I-Thou" relationship, there are infinite possibilities.

"It-It" & "It-Thou"

What if you don't consider *yourself* an "I"? What if your authentic self doesn't exist in the relationship? Do you treat yourself as an object? Are you only an "It"?

Part of that "I-Thou" experience is the "I" part. It could be that we have never been treated like a "Thou" before. Maybe growing up, we were treated as objects by our parents. Maybe we were treated as objects in school or at work or in past relationships. The hard reality is that if we have been treated like that our whole life, we may not even consider ourselves an "I".

This can lead to having experiences like "It-It" where we don't consider ourselves as anything important and we think the same about everyone else. We treat our kids this way, our parents, our friends, and our colleagues. It's a dog-eat-dog world and everyone has to fend for themselves.

Or maybe we have an "It-Thou" experience where we treat our partner and others as worthy and important. We consider their needs, their opinions, and their existence as more important than our own. Our feelings and desires don't matter. We are just thankful to get to be in their lives. We are content to be treated as an object as long as it makes them happy, and they keep us around.

Rollo May, an American psychologist, once stated that until we have the "I am" experience, no therapy or process can help us feel happy or better about our lives. We must be part of the equation for any kind of real relationship to happen. Otherwise, what are we really doing?

Your Personal Journey:
1. Can you imagine the kind of union where both of you disappear into bliss? Can you imagine it in your mind? Can you feel it in your soul?
2. What kind of relationships do you prefer? Loving co-existence? Passionate eros? Something else?
3. Can you relate to Martin Buber's "I-Thou" experience? Who do you have this kind of connection with now? Or with whom have you had this in the past?
4. Do you consider yourself an "I" in your relationships? If not, where does this come from? What experiences need to be looked at to bring you back into the game as the beautiful "Thou" that you truly are?

SECTION II

The Masculine & Feminine Dynamics

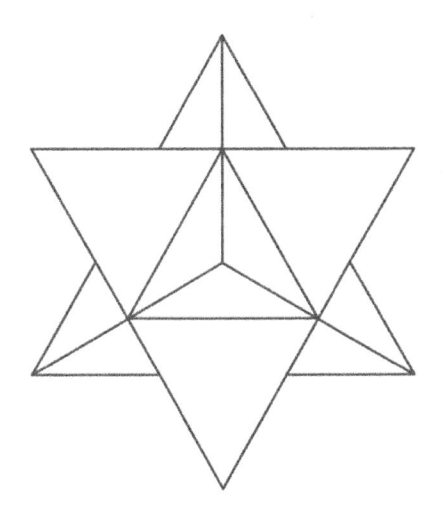

Chapter 4
Giving & Receiving

He arrived at my apartment with a bag of groceries and said, "You relax. I'm going to make the most delicious dinner!" He proceeded to take out the groceries, start chopping vegetables, and heat up the stove. Then he poured me a drink and asked me to go sit on the couch beside the island (my place was all open-concept).

I put on some music and happily watched him. He chit-chatted while he cooked, every so often looking up at me to smile. As I sat there watching him, I was struck by how happy he was. He wasn't doing this because he had to or was trying to impress me. He seemed to truly want to do this.

While the steaks were cooking, he set the table, moved my drink to the table, and then motioned for me to go and sit there. When I tried to offer to help, he pretended to be angry and said, "No! You just relax."

At this point, something started to break inside of me. I had taken care of everyone my whole life. I'd taken care of my kids, my husband, my family, and anyone else who came along. I had fantasized about having a man in my life who loved to do this kind of thing—to give in total joy—but truthfully, some part of me had given up hope.

As he walked toward me with plates of delicious food, tears started to roll down my cheeks. I had no idea just how much I had desired this. I had no idea how much this meant to me.

He looked surprised and said, "Are you crying?"

"Yes... I can't tell you how much I appreciate this."

We hugged tightly for a long time and, lucky for me, there would be many more times like this to come.

There can be great joy in giving and great joy in receiving. The bliss of union happens when we give something to someone who truly desires what we are giving. Similarly, when we need something, there is great joy in receiving it from someone who truly wants to give it. The person receiving will naturally appreciate the gift, and this appreciation is exactly what fills the giver's heart.

The Act of Giving

> *"It's not how much we give,
> but how much love we put into the giving."*
> MOTHER TERESA

The energy of giving is masculine and receiving is feminine. In most situations, this has nothing to do with gender or whether we identify as the masculine or feminine partner. It is simply the dynamic of giving something to someone who needs it. The key is to understand the difference between giving in connection versus in separation.

In connection, giving could look like a parent (masculine) feeding a hungry child (feminine), a teacher (masculine) sharing with students (feminine), a donor (masculine) giving to a charity (feminine), a healthcare practitioner (masculine) helping a patient (feminine), or a masculine lover kissing and caressing their feminine partner.

In separation, this might be a parent feeding a child something they don't want, someone telling you to eat something even though you are full, a teacher presenting information regardless of whom they are talking to, students not open to the teachings, someone giving money to another with strings attached, a person in need not accepting help, a doctor prescribing something without considering the wisdom of the patient, having sex with your partner as an object, or someone helping another only to make themselves feel better.

We have done all of these things for millennia without realizing that there were other options. We knew that they didn't feel good but we didn't know how else to interact. These things happening in separation is why relationships have often been so difficult and filled with hard feelings.

THE SPIRIT OF GIVING

What could giving feel like? Let's imagine that we are a magnet. We have both masculine and feminine within us. Through the feminine energy, we receive from others, loved ones, the sunshine, and God until we are overflowing. Through the masculine, we give that energy out to the world.

This is why there can be so much joy in giving. It is literally loving energy flowing through us and out to others. Of course, if we have struggled to receive in the past, or if what we have received has been painful, giving may be difficult. So, if this is the case, our journey may begin with opening ourselves to receiving, which we'll talk more about soon.

Giving is the look on your child's face when you have given them a gift that they really wanted but weren't expecting. Giving is anonymously paying for the person's coffee behind you in the drive-thru and driving away smiling. Giving is massaging your lover and feeling so incredibly grateful that they trust you to let you caress their skin this way.

Giving feels wonderful and not only makes the receiver happy, it fills the soul of the giver as well.

So, what are some examples of giving?

DOING KIND THINGS FOR OTHERS

My partner making me a beautiful dinner is a wonderful example of this. This is the act of doing things that are unasked for and you know that the other person will appreciate it.

I remember one year at University, I was particularly broke. I was putting myself through school and had hit one of those months where all I had was wilted celery in my fridge and wouldn't start working again for a couple of months (I was in a cooperative program).

One day, my grandfather came to visit me on campus. He was a very quiet man—an Anglican minister—who was very kind, didn't say a whole lot, but was loved by everyone he came into contact with. I had shown him around the campus, had lunch with him, and was walking him to his car as he slipped an envelope into my hand.

He looked at me with a twinkle in his eyes and said, "Open it later. It's for you."

Well, after he drove away, I opened the envelope to find a crisp hundred-dollar bill. I nearly cried. That was like a million dollars to me. That would get me through till my next work term.

This was a wonderful masculine gesture of giving.

Helping Others

The most important thing we need to know about helping is that we read the other person and give them what they need.

A while ago, my son needed help moving. This puts him in the feminine. I asked him, "What do you need? How can I help?" He replied, "Well, it would just be nice to have someone to help carry the boxes up the stairs and load the truck and all that." So, I gave him what he needed. We loaded boxes and we had a joyful day together.

What if, instead, I had responded with, "Well, how about I'll bring you lunch at noon?"

I am giving something that I want to give because I don't want to carry boxes. He might accept the lunch, but no connection will be made in the interaction. He didn't receive what he needed. He didn't need food. He needed help moving boxes. It isn't that it's wrong to bring food. Maybe my knees couldn't take the stairs. That's okay. However, it is possible that he wasn't even planning on stopping for lunch. Maybe he just wanted to get into his new place. Knowing my son, he would have stopped and eaten the food I had brought out of obligation. This isn't evil but it doesn't create any kind of union or connection at all.

Volunteering

Giving our time, expertise, or money is a wonderful gift for those who need them. This could be a local non-profit, a friend, or a stranger.

The key here is to choose something that gives you joy. We have had a lot of training in the past that it is expected of us to give to charities. We are told that this makes us good people or upstanding members of the community. However, these reasons do not create union with those we want to help. Obligatory giving simply fulfills a lacking within ourselves and creates no connection at all in the world.

Instead, if you love animals, volunteer at the shelter. If you love music, give your money or expertise to the local symphony group. If you have a passion for helping those who are homeless, volunteer at a soup kitchen.

The key is that our hearts are involved. We want every experience to open us up to others.

Giving Services to Others

I have a good friend who is a chiropractor and one of the gentlest men I've ever met. After he read my book "Tantric Intimacy," I happened to go in for a treatment. We chit-chatted for a while before he said, "You know, I think I have to work on being more masculine in life. I think I'm pretty passive overall."

This gave me so much pause. Although he was a very quiet, peaceful man (stereotypically opposite of what we might think of as masculine), he spent his days serving others (masculine). However, I also observed his incredible balance of the masculine and feminine. When he talked to his patients during their sessions, he really listened to whatever was going on in their lives—to the point that his waiting room was often backed up as each session went on far longer than planned.

When he worked with you, he was incredibly conscious. You knew that he was present and listening within for guidance. And his services were excellent.

It is possible that he was referring to how he acted in relationships—which is outside of my knowledge of him—but it was fascinating to connect how masculine (and feminine) he was all day long, in perfect balance, which perhaps contributed to how incredibly peaceful I felt around him.

The Role of the Receiver

There is often a lot of confusion around receiving. Sometimes, we think it means that we don't do anything. There are even negative connotations around being the one in need, and yet, there are times when we all need something. It might be help, kind words, a massage, or a glass of water. It's normal to have needs, and it is wonderful when the Universe provides for us.

THE SPIRIT OF RECEIVING

Oh, the gratitude of receiving. When someone does something kind for us, we completely receive it in every cell of our body. When we receive what we need, we just feel thankful. When we can openly receive, we feel very lucky. This is how we are nourished by others and the world. This is opening ourselves and saying "YES!" to life.

When we fully receive this abundance, our whole being expands. The walls around us disappear and we happily merge with the person giving to us and our surroundings. We breathe more deeply. We feel a wonderful sense of inner joy and true belonging.

Appreciation

A big part of receiving is appreciating the gift. However, genuine appreciation can be a challenge because we are often taught to pretend that we appreciate things whether we do or not. We are taught that this is "being polite." Sometimes, people might only give to us for the appreciation that their ego will receive. They may give because they want the "admiration of others," which makes genuine appreciation seldom happen for them. So, this idea of appreciation needs some fine-tuning.

As a receiver, we don't owe the giver appreciation. This kind of expectation happens when there's separation. This is when someone has given you something that they didn't really want to give you and is now demanding appreciation for it—like wanting a gold star for a job well-done. Perhaps someone has given you something that you neither asked for nor wanted and then demands appreciation. But how can we genuinely appreciate something that was neither wanted nor needed.

This goes awry because the giver has an agenda. They aren't giving in joy. This creates a feeling of being forced on both sides. It is uncomfortable for everyone. Appreciation is impossible because whatever they gave wasn't desired, or it created so much drama, it wasn't worth it.

Instead, let's imagine that you mention to your partner that you're thinking of getting a bookcase for your room, but you're having a hard time finding one that has the right measurements. Maybe your birthday is coming up, and your partner secretly goes on a hunt for the perfect bookcase. On the day of your birthday, you come home from work to see a beautiful bookcase in your room. You are genuinely filled with appreciation. You can't believe they went to all that trouble. You can't believe that they were able to keep it a secret. You throw your arms around them in the warmest embrace, filling them and the room with blissful appreciation.

Maybe someone cooks your favourite meal or takes you to your favourite restaurant. If you simply eat the meal and go on with your day, hopefully, they will still have enjoyed planning this gift and making it happen. However, if you look at them with genuine appreciation, this is where union occurs. This is where happiness overflows, and you both feel wonderfully connected to each other.

Appreciation in sexual intimacy is when you totally relax into the touch of your lover. You are genuinely happy to be with them. You love how they touch, kiss, and caress you. This isn't put on or faked in any way. You are genuinely enjoying the pleasure. As you relax into receiving, your partner will feel it in your body's responses and your kisses. The beautiful feeling of happiness you emanate flows back into your partner, and the wonderful cycle of energy builds and builds between you.

Asking for Help

It is a great thing to know that we can always ask for help. We soon learn that we are not alone, and we can often find much better solutions after a good discussion with a friend.

When I'm upset, I will usually call a friend or one of my kids. Some people tend to withdraw when they are upset, but I am more of a verbal processor. I'll call people and say, "Hey, can we talk? Here's what's going on. Here's what I'm thinking. What do you think? Do I sound crazy? I'd love to know your thoughts."

They will share their perceptions of what they hear. They don't normally give me advice, but they do share what comes to them. I ask, and they give. We are in union. They don't expect me to follow their advice. There are no strings attached to the conversation in any way. I asked a question, and they answered. The communication is complete. The masculine and feminine joined together to help me sort through a difficult patch.

Becoming Interdependent

A friend of mine is a staunchly independent woman. She came to Canada as a young adult and learned quickly how to do whatever she needed to do. She also learned that reaching out to others didn't always work out the way she hoped. It was way easier for her to just become totally independent.

One day, while walking across a city street, she was hit by a car and her ankle was broken. She couldn't drive. She couldn't walk. When she first got her cast on, she could barely make it up a single step. She had no idea what she was going to do.

She did have friends around her that she could call on — if she could allow herself to. But now, of course, she had to. She had no choice. The Universe often has a way of helping us learn whatever we deeply desire.

Her aunt and uncle happily took her in to take care of her. They set her up in a comfy chair. They brought her food, drinks, and anything else she needed. Initially, she was dying inside. To just receive without giving anything back was nearly killing her. However, deep down, she was also relieved. She was so thankful that they were happy to do it. She couldn't believe how kind they were to her. The experience seriously changed her.

She realized that she had great people in her life. She realized that people loved her, and they loved having her around. Even strangers were more than happy to help her into restaurants or in tough spaces that she couldn't navigate on her own.

Kind people were everywhere. She had never realized that before.

The Even-Steven Challenge

Even-steven is an old English phrase that means not being owed anything and not owing anything. If I borrow money and repay you, we are now "even-steven." It is defined as a mutually beneficial trade or a tied score in an athletic contest.

However, we often bring this idea into many aspects of our lives which can confuse our ideas of giving and receiving. It makes us think that if someone gives to us, then we must give back in equal measure. This might work in business and sports but it has nothing to do with union.

Instead, let's imagine that when someone needs something and we have it to give, we give it to them. This is the end of the experience. No one is keeping tabs. The receiver does not owe the giver anything. The giver simply gave something they had to someone who needed it. The "transaction" is complete.

Maybe you go to a friend's house and they make you a coffee. You sit for hours chatting and pondering life together, and then you head home. This experience is complete. You could invite your friend to your house one day if you want, but you don't have to do it just because they invited you over. You don't owe them anything. They gave, you received, and you both had a wonderful time together.

Perhaps this idea comes from a scarcity mentality — that if I give you something, then you must return the favour because now I will have to go without. Or maybe it comes from the hoarding of wealth and material things, and we are afraid to part with anything. Therefore, if I give you something, you'd better either give it back to me or give me something of equal value.

When we have children, they need food, shelter, protection, and love. As parents, we give this to them. The transaction is complete. The children don't owe us anything. As parents, we filled true needs of the beings that we brought into the Earth. However, this even-steven idea has even crept into our parent-child relationships where some people believe that their children owe them something because they had to give so much as parents. You can just feel the weight, the guilt trips, the sadness, and the separation in this mentality. There is no union. No happiness. No joy in giving or receiving. Just separation and heartache that often builds upon itself and comes out in aggressive and passive aggressive ways for both the parents and children for most of their time together.

The key is to only give when our desire is simply for the other person to receive. That's it.

On a similar note, when someone gives us a compliment, we must receive it without giving it back. If someone comes up to you and says, "Wow, you are such a great person!" and you reply, "You're a great person, too!", you basically just zeroed out the whole experience. Their compliment meant nothing. They were giving you something, and you just returned it to them. Sometimes we even fish for compliments this way—giving a compliment to someone so that they will say something nice to us—a way of using this even-steven idea to get praise from others.

Imagine this sexually. If we do the even-steven thing, the energy just goes back and forth. I do this for you, and you return it. You do this for me, and I return it. You are like two masculine energies playing tennis. This can still be exciting and full of sexual pleasure. But you can't have the enjoyment of fully receiving because you're always thinking about how you're going to give it back. This isn't union. This is two separate people doing things to each other.

Instead, when the masculine partner fully gives, and every ounce of the feminine receives, energy flows between you. There is no even-steven. Each is contributing a different kind of energy that amp each other up. This is where the magic happens. This is where energy flows and nourishes each person. No even-steven ideas apply.

The Unhealthy Flip: The Serving Feminine

Because of our patriarchal history, the idea that the masculine is the giving, nurturing energy, and the feminine receives, is often confusing. In many families, the men were truly in the masculine by working to provide for their families and protecting their loved ones. Yet, within the intimate relationship of the couple, the men were often in the feminine role of receiving, and the women were in the masculine role of serving.

MASCULINE & FEMININE DYNAMICS

When I was first dating my husband, I would watch the men sit at the kitchen table while the women ran around serving coffee, fetching the ketchup, and getting refills. In this case, the men were in the feminine receiving, and the women were in full masculine giving.

The women would plan the events and holidays and organize the children, while the men rested after a long day at work. Yes, this may not be the way it is now, and there have always been exceptions to the rule, but by and large, this was the division of labour in the home for a long time.

The women served the men. The women were in the masculine role. The men were in the feminine. This is similar to the master-slave archetype where the master would consider himself to be in the "powerful" masculine and the slave in the "weak" feminine. But, in actuality, the slave is doing for the master and is, therefore, in the masculine, while the master receives in the feminine. We might call the one serving being in the false-feminine and the master in the false-masculine.

This flip damages both parties. It is not a natural polarity and connection. It is created through this domination paradigm and through the preferences of the men who were once in charge. The false-feminine has no choice and is not considered except in how they can serve the false-masculine.

This exhausts those in the false-feminine and doesn't allow them to live in their true powerful nature, and although those in the false-masculine might feel like they are in the power-seat, this is actually totally disempowering for them which leads to drama in intimate relationships, power struggles, and impotence in life.

This is one of the greatest flipped paradigms that we need to release in order to embrace the merging and union of the masculine and feminine.[1]

---

[1] We will discuss this more in Chapter 18 where we look at common masculine-feminine archetypes.

Removing the Idea of "Give & Take"

Sometimes we come to a place in our life where we just don't want to give anymore. Sometimes we are exhausted. Sometimes we don't have whatever is needed to give. But often, the problem is that we have been surrounded by "takers" who have exhausted our desire to give another thing.

Taking is not the same as receiving. Taking is going and getting what you want. Receiving is being an empty vessel and allowing yourself to be filled. When someone takes from you, you have no joy in the giving because it wasn't voluntary. They just took something from you whether you had it to give or not. This is acting in total separation.

Adam Grant wrote a great book called *Give and Take.* He talks about how there are people who are natural "givers," and others whom he calls "takers." When you are a natural giver, you love to give. You get great joy in giving, and you don't need others to give back to you. There are no strings attached. You aren't giving out of obligation—just the true joy of giving.

If you end up connected to someone who is a taker, that person just takes and takes like a black hole. Maybe it's your emotional strength that they lean on, and you tell yourself it's okay because they've been hurt a lot in the past. Or maybe it's financial, but you're okay because you've got money, and you feel very grateful for your abundance. Maybe it's gifts, kind gestures, car rides, touch, or attention.

This taking can go on for a long time, and then, a day will come when you don't want to give anymore. You have the feeling of being "bled dry". As much as you don't give to receive appreciation, the fact that there is no appreciation at all is quite disheartening. The problem is that these are not "give and receive" relationships. They are "give and take" transactions. The taker is more like a parasite feeding rather than someone receiving something they need.

Soon, the giver will start to separate from the taker, and become a "matcher." A matcher only gives as much as the other person gives. It is a self-preservation mechanism for natural givers when they are connected to a taker. That taker could be a boss, partner, friend, child, or family member. These are the people we start to keep tabs with because if we don't, we will end up very empty and have nothing left to give to ourselves or anyone else.

However, keeping track takes all the fun out of giving. You can't just give from your heart anymore. Everything must be calculated. Luckily, we seldom remain a "matcher" for very long because we soon realize that there is nothing to match. Our taker never gives anything to us. Instead, they are more likely to leave, say that we don't love them enough, and go find another giver to fulfill their needs.

If we want to have a give-and-receive relationship, then we have to find a different friend or partner. However, if we have been surrounded by takers our whole life, it is often quite a journey to find these people and truly trust them.

Challenges in Giving

Giving Without Strings Attached

Sometimes we give things because we want to get something back. We might give someone a compliment expecting that they'll say that you look great, too. I give you a gift so that you can give me a gift. We do something for someone so that they'll do something for us later. Or maybe we give something to someone, and they simply owe us. We will decide how we will even the score later.

This kind of giving is manipulation. It might not seem like it because it is so normalized in our families, relationships, friendships, and careers. Families have been keeping score for centuries, but this is not the kind of connection we are seeking.

This also becomes very difficult on the receiving side because if people have always given to us in order to get something back, it won't take too many times before we don't want to receive anything from anyone. We would rather go without than be indebted to them. This creates a greater separation and even less interaction than before. We can easily start creating a life where we are more like an island unto ourselves. It seems easier that way. No debts to others. Just the freedom to live as we want.

Giving From Our Heart

We want to be careful that we are truly giving from our hearts.

Let's say that you are passionate about helping those who are homeless. Maybe you know someone who was homeless, or maybe you were once homeless and you want to give back. You require nothing of those you are helping. You simply want to give. That is the end of it. That is the end of the experience.

I personally give to certain charities, and I get quite upset when they send me gifts in the mail to thank me for giving them money. I don't want a gift. I want all of my donation to go to the people they're helping. That is my only reason for giving.

But what if we are giving for other reasons? Imagine a scenario where someone gives money to someone living on the street and then says "Make sure you buy food with this!" Or they take a picture of themselves "giving" to this person. Is this really a gift? Or was it an excuse to feel better about themselves? Or maybe we give money to a family member when they need it. We now figure that they owe us because of what we have done for them. None of this is union, happiness, or bliss. It is manipulation, opportunism, and, sometimes, the actions of a guilty conscience.

This is the challenge when we are taught to give because we should and not genuinely from our hearts.

Maybe we think that we should volunteer at an old age home and read to the seniors as opposed to simply wanting to read to the elderly. These are very different experiences. Can you imagine the difference in the experience of those older people when someone is reading to them because they genuinely want to versus out of obligation?

In the first scenario, the readers might genuinely have great respect for our elders and just want to share with them. Maybe one of the residents says, "Thank you so much for coming down here. I'm sure you're very busy." You can happily respond, "Are you kidding? I love this. I love this book, I love reading, and I get to share it with you. This is awesome for me!" Imagine how that feels to the one receiving.

Then, we have the second scenario where I figure that I should do two hours a week doing charity work because that is what good people do. So, I choose reading to seniors because it's easy, it's inside, and it fits into my schedule. I go to the seniors' home, go through the motions, and secretly hope the clock moves quickly. Imagine the poor person listening. Deep down they know that you don't want to be there. You may end up making them feel like they are just a charity case.

The key is that giving and receiving must always be a win-win, or else, there is no real connection or joy. If we're helping someone, and we believe that it is only for the receiver's benefit, there's a high chance that they are not benefiting at all. Only our ego is benefitting and we are telling ourselves a story about how much we helped them and what a good person we are when, in fact, they are no further ahead and, in the end, might even feel a little bit worse about themselves and their situation.

Challenges in Receiving

There is also a great challenge in receiving due to the domination paradigm. Receiving can feel scary because, historically, those in the feminine (children, women, workers, students) have seldom received what they desired. But, no matter what, we were trained to be polite and say "thank you" no matter what was given to us.

We also know that there are often strings attached to receiving that make us want to withdraw from many connections with people—especially family—making us feel very alone.

Because of this separation between the giver and the receiver, many twists have developed over the millennia—passive aggression, fierce independence, becoming a "taker", becoming a people-pleaser and doormat, and many more. So, we need to look at what healthy receiving is alongside the challenges we have had in the past.

It is Okay to Receive

In many societies, only the masculine is considered important. Only the giver is valued. They are considered the strong ones. They are the ones with the money, food, power, advice, or talent. They are the important ones in any interaction. The one who receives is just the one "in need" or listening or "just lying there, not doing anything." (Notice how often we use the word "just" when describing the feminine). The feminine's importance is disregarded and can be considered quite lowly.

So, our ego may struggle with this receiver role. We may not understand the value of being a true listener or a great audience. We may not honour the feminine within that has great wisdom and strength. We don't allow ourselves to have needs that could be happily fulfilled by others. We may not understand the strength it takes to admit our struggles and ask for help.

Many people also struggle to receive in intimacy. Maybe deep down, they don't believe that they deserve pleasure. Some feel badly because they think that being the receiver means "just lying there", but this couldn't be further from the truth. The feminine's body is actually like a radio receiver, taking the masculine energy given, and broadcasting it as it flows through both bodies, creating pure ecstasy for everyone.

We All Deserve to Receive

Sometimes we believe that we don't deserve to receive anything. Many religions taught us that we are sinful by birth, our thoughts are wrong, we must work for salvation, and even if we do everything right, we are still "sinful in the eyes of God." This deep training makes joyful receiving a great challenge.

In many cultures, if you are born a girl, you are less important than boys. If you were born a certain ethnicity, there may be racist people around who treat you as being less than them. If we do not line up with the expectations of others, they may shame us and make us feel even worse about ourselves. All of these things can truly leave us in a place where we have a hard time receiving anything at all.

I once worked with a man who was having sexual issues. I loved working with him because he had such a kind heart. In life, he was a true giver. He just gave and gave and gave. He worked with disadvantaged children. He was that guy that everybody loved — the fun guy, the kind guy, the guy who was always there for everyone.

However, he absolutely couldn't receive. Even in the work that he and I were doing together, big changes were happening within him, and he would try to give me the credit. He would say that everything was happening because of my "magic." We would talk about all the inner work that he was doing, but no matter how many nice things I said to him, he would just bounce them back to me.

At one point, his homework was that he wasn't allowed to bounce back compliments. He had to learn to receive them. When he went to work the next day, one of his colleagues came up to him and said, "You know, that work you did with the group the other day was so profound. I've had so many kids come up to me and tell me how much it touched them."

He didn't know what to say. He went through all the scripts in his head like "Oh well, anyone could have done it." or "You could have done it, too." or "Those kids were on the brink of breakthrough anyway." But he wasn't allowed to say any of those. He had to just receive this beautiful truth about himself. There were no strings attached to what his colleague was saying. She was simply giving him truthful feedback on something he'd done.

When he went home that night and saw his kids, they had things they wanted to thank him for. He took a deep breath and said, "You're welcome. It was a pleasure." He actually allowed it in.

The next time he came to me, he was aghast. He realized that people gave to him all the time. People were constantly kind to him. They were always doing things or wanting to do things for him, and he'd never allowed it.

Part of his history was that he had been raised in a tough part of town, surrounded by alcoholism and physical abuse. He had had to block his heart from receiving because, at a very young age, he learned that it was dangerous to receive. It was dangerous to be open, and if you did receive something now, you would owe someone something later that you may not want to repay in the way that they want.

Make Sure You Want What You're Being Given

I work with a lot of women (although this applies to men, as well) who believe that they struggle to receive. They imagine this to be a character flaw. They say, "I'm just not good at receiving. I must have blocks to others or something. Maybe it was my childhood or the way my ex-partner treated me." The next question I ask is, "Are you good at receiving things that you actually want? Or are you just not good at receiving things that you don't want?"

This is an important question because when we are in separation and are perpetually being given things that we don't want, we are not going to want to receive them. It is very simple. It doesn't mean we aren't good receivers. It just means that we are discerning.

Imagine this in intimacy. Your partner wants to have sex with you. At that moment, you're not in the mood. If your partner is connected to you, they will happily do something else like offer to cuddle. If they aren't connected to you, they may get defensive and say, "Why don't you want to have sex? Are you in a bad mood? Aren't you attracted to me anymore? Do you even love me?"

Of course, they are not reading you at all. You are simply the object of their desire. They want to have sex, and you're the one they have sex with. You're not a human with interesting things going on inside. You're not a being with desires, drives, and emotions. You are just something that they want to do something to. So, it's quite natural to not want to receive this because you simply don't desire it at that moment.

We have a similar problem with unsolicited advice. This is something that many people take great joy in giving, but it is rarely wanted by the receiver. Yet the one giving it feels very good about themselves. Essentially, the giver has simplified your life in a way that they can see a clear solution and are thrilled they can share it with you. This could be from someone who genuinely loves you and is worried about you or from someone who isn't so nice and is trying to make you feel small.

Regardless, neither bit of advice is asked for. And even the one who is doing it out of "love" is not reading their recipient. Their recipient has not asked. Of course, when the person doesn't take the unwanted guidance, they are criticized as being "unwilling to listen," stubborn, willful, or too ignorant to take excellent advice.

If we want to be in union with someone, then we need to give them something they are seeking. If a question arises within someone, a receptor is opened that can now be filled. But without that receptor, even if you have the best advice in the world, there is nowhere for it to go.

If we truly honoured and tried to read the feminine, we would know that they were asking what 1+4 is, and we would stop screaming "Purple!" at them, wondering why they aren't "receiving our good advice."

Your Personal Journey:

STRENGTHENING THE FEMININE

1. Are you comfortable receiving? Are there certain people from whom you enjoy receiving? Are there others from whom you don't? What is the difference?
2. Do you believe that you deserve to receive? If not, where does this come from?
3. Are you comfortable saying "no" to things you don't want to receive? Advice? Help? Sexual advances?
4. Are you afraid to receive sometimes because there are strings attached?

STRENGTHENING THE MASCULINE

1. Do you experience joy in giving? Are there certain people to whom you love giving? Are there others that you don't?
2. Do you give with no strings attached? If there are sometimes strings, where does this pattern come from?
3. Do you only give out of joy? Or do you often give out of expectation? Were you raised with this "Even-Steven" idea that if I give to you, you will give the equivalent back?
4. In romantic relationships, how do you love to give?

MASCULINE & FEMININE DYNAMICS

Chapter 5
Talking & Listening

In 1999, I went through a healing crisis. This is when I met Jim, my first spiritual teacher. When I would go for sessions with him, the number one thing we did was talk.

As he would talk, I was transfixed. It was like every word he said was exactly the medicine I needed at that moment. After he would complete a thought, we might sit in silence as I let what he'd said sink in. As a question arose, I would withdraw from the listening mode to form my question.

Eyes locked on each other, he would listen to my question, think for a minute, and answer me.

He was the wisest person I had ever met. He felt like he was about 500 years old, so I listened to him intently. The crazy thing is that I know that I heard much more than the words that he spoke. In many spiritual traditions, they speak of receiving a transmission from the guru. This is what I believe was happening. It was like, through our connection, a channel locked in place between us, and whatever I needed to know flooded into me.

A kind of communion happened. A loving trust. A true union of souls.

Communion in Communication

Talking is masculine and listening is feminine. This is one of the most common examples of the giving-receiving dynamic because it is how we communicate with each other.

First, let's look at the word "communication." Breaking it down, it comes from the words "to commune," "to merge," and "to come together." What if every time we spoke to another person, the only reason we did so was to commune with them and draw closer together? Through talking and listening, we have an opportunity for connection. Imagine how differently we would communicate if that was always our intention.

You may have someone in your life with whom you communicate this way. When you talk, they listen, and when they talk, you listen because you're interested in their perspective. This is union. These kinds of conversations can go on for hours and hours without any awareness of time passing.

Then there are conversations where both people are in the masculine. I say something, and then you say something. You say something, and then I say something. No one is really listening. It is more like a debate or a tennis match. Arguments have this dynamic. Everyone is wanting the other person to hear them. Sometimes, people are simply used to being the ones speaking, so the conversation is just a series of statements and stories from each person. No one is listening. It is just statements and stories filling the air.

There are other times when you both seem to be in the feminine. Everyone is waiting for someone to say something. This can be a very peaceful way for two people to sit together. There is nothing wrong with this, but for our discussion, there is no magnetic connection because they are not really listening to the other. They are both simply whole in their own selves. As soon as one steps into the masculine and says something to the other, their energies are now focused on each other and connection happens.

The Role of Speaker

*"If you talk to a man in a language he understands,
that goes to his head.
If you talk to him in his language, that goes to his heart"*
NELSON MANDELA

THE SPIRIT OF SPEAKING

We want to bring a new kind of awareness to our conversations because we have centuries of unconscious, disconnected communication behind us. There are many situations where someone is just talking, and it doesn't even matter if anyone is listening. Sometimes, we just talk because we love the story we're telling. Sometimes, we talk out of nervousness or because we are uncomfortable with silence. Sometimes, we speak in order to silence another person or to intimidate them. Other times, it is just mindless chatter not needing to land anywhere, just speaking whatever stream of consciousness enters our mind.

The question is, "Do any of these situations lead to a deeper connection?" Unfortunately, most lead to more separation than before the words were spoken. So, how do we change how we communicate?

The first thing to be aware of is our intention. If our intention is to intimidate or overpower the other person using words, then this is exactly what will happen. If our intention is to make ourselves seem smart, then this will form what we say. If we truly want to connect with the other person, then we will choose our words based on the person we are speaking to.

This is where we must remember that the masculine is born out of the feminine. We speak based on what the listener desires to hear. Have they asked a question? Have they signed up for a class with you to learn something? Would they like your thoughts on something? Are you brainstorming together in order to find a new idea?

So, what do we need to know in order to connect with others in this way?

Meeting People Where They Are

> *"If you can't explain it to a six-year-old, you don't understand it yourself."*
> ALBERT EINSTEIN

Healthy communicators are not only articulate with their words, they are also fully aware of their listeners and adapt to them. There are obvious examples of this when we are travelling and speaking to people for whom English is their second language. We naturally slow down and choose simpler words that are more likely to be in their vocabulary and still be able to say everything we want to say.

However, for people who speak the same language, we often aren't so careful. Maybe we studied English Literature in school and have a wide vocabulary that is not commonly used. If we use this vocabulary with people who have not studied English Literature extensively, they will not understand what we are saying, and a distance will form between us.

Maybe we are lawyers, doctors, economists, or computer technicians who regularly use jargon in our work that others don't use. Maybe we are particularly enthralled with Eastern religion and have picked up many spiritual terms referring to concepts seldom expressed in the West. If we use our specific jargon with everyone, many people will not know what we are saying or understand the depths of the words we are using. So, no real communication is possible.

Sometimes we love to "speak over the heads" of others because it makes us feel smart. There may even be times when it is done intentionally to intimidate the listener and make them feel dumb. And sometimes, it isn't done to be mean or intimidating. We simply might talk about things with our colleagues and community so much that we lose touch with which words in our vocabulary are not understood by those outside the jargon of our community.

This is why it is important to stay aware of our listener at all times. If we begin to describe something, and we can feel a distance forming, then we must adapt our language to them.

It is important to note that this isn't "talking down to someone." Just because someone else doesn't use the same vocabulary that we use doesn't make them less intelligent. They simply use a different language than we do.

It all comes back to our intention for speaking. If our intention is for the listener to understand what we are saying, then the only logical thing to do is to speak in a way that truly reaches them.

I have always loved the above Einstein quote because, within the domination paradigm, language has often been used to dominate others. Within that paradigm, the masculine is never wrong. If someone explains something, and the listener doesn't understand, it is the fault of the listener. They are considered not smart enough, not a good listener, or simply unable to understand. There is no responsibility placed on the speaker at all.

Yet the words of Einstein say something different. Imagine instead that the speaker has half the responsibility for the interaction. Yes, the listener must truly be listening. They can't be distracted, intoxicated, or not paying attention. But assuming the listener is truly listening, the speaker's only responsibility is to speak in a way that they can hear.

We simply communicate to connect with the listener. No one is above the other. There is no power play of intelligence—just the desire to deeply connect through verbal communication.

Staying Focused on Our Listener

If we love to talk, we may need a transitional period where we have to become aware of how we speak to others. Are we just telling a story for ourselves, or does the listener truly want to hear it? Are we just filling the silence because it's unnerving to us?

Another thing that can happen is that the speaker can head off on an irrelevant tangent. When this happens, the listener will naturally disengage because energetically, they know that what's being spoken isn't really for them. The speaker is now talking to themselves. However, we have been taught at home, and especially at school, to pretend like we are listening, even though we are not interested at all. This perpetuates the speaker's complete disconnection from the listener.

So, it may take a concerted effort for you, as a speaker, to remain focused on the person listening. Isn't it strange that we have to learn to speak in a way that our listener can hear us? Theoretically, the listener is the only reason that we are speaking. Why else would we be talking?

Being a Listener

> *"Deep listening is the kind of listening that can help relieve the suffering of another person."*
> THICH NHAT HANH

How to Be a Great Listener

This is only possible when you want to hear what is being spoken. If you are with someone who is only talking about things you aren't interested in, you will not want to receive what they are saying any more than you would eat the sandwich offered to you when you aren't hungry.

Instead, let's assume that the reason they are speaking is for connection, understanding, or for you to learn something. The key to being a listener isn't just sitting there and being passive. It is actively listening. You are paying full attention. You are receiving, absorbing, and processing all that is being said.

The funny thing about this is that if we are truly interested, we don't have to tell ourselves to pay attention or be intrigued. We *are* intrigued. The intrigue is the foundation of the conversation. That's the reason it's happening.

However, this isn't always the case. So, let's look at some challenges that we may come across.

Forced Listening Doesn't Create Connection

Being a listener can be a challenge because we have been trained from a very young age to listen in separation. We had to listen without any conscious connection to how we felt. We were often in total separation—from the speaker and ourselves. In my childhood, children were to be seen and not heard. How often did we hear, "Just listen! Be quiet and listen to me!"

In school, we are forced to listen whether we are interested or not. It is drilled into us. You must sit there and pretend that you are listening. You can't fall asleep. You can't show that you are bored, and you're not allowed to leave. This training begins at a very impressionable young age and continues for at least thirteen years—our most formative years.

This is dangerous because we don't learn how to send signals to the person who is speaking to us. We don't know how to communicate that this is not what we want to listen to. If we said that in school, we would be punished. This is very deep training woven into our psyche.

This is important to unearth because forcing ourselves to listen can drain our energy and even create a kind of depression. And it's not only listening—this dynamic will show up in all of our giving-receiving experiences. In the same way that we feel that we must listen and suffer silently, we will also feel that we have to receive whatever someone is giving us because it is the same energy dynamic.

The Speaker Is Speaking for Themselves

What if we are sitting with someone who is a disconnected speaker and is telling you the same story for the fifth time or talking about their most recent vacation or a show that they're watching, and you're not interested in any of it? It can be quite a challenge to gently shift the conversation toward something you truly want to engage with.

If they're telling you a story you've heard before, you can be honest in a kind way and say, "Yes, you've told me this story before. It's wonderful." Or if they are showing you photos of their trip, and there's no getting out of it, you can actively think about questions you could ask that would have interesting answers. We are so accustomed to being passive listeners, we have forgotten that there might be some very interesting side notes to these trips by which we could be intrigued. Do we want to know about the food? The culture? Their favourite area? A place they would return to? Sports? If we ask questions about topics that we are personally interested in, the whole conversation will become very dynamic. They really want to share about their trip. We just have to think about the aspects that we'd be interested in and steer the conversation that way. (Of course, the first step is being honest when they ask you if you want to see pictures from their trip. If you say "yes" out of politeness, then we know what's coming. Instead, we could say, "I'd rather not look at the pictures, but I'd love to hear about the parts that were meaningful for you.")

If they are telling you about a show they're watching, you can say, "Wow. I've never seen that show. What is it that draws you to it? Have there been moments in it that have affected you?"

The key is to break out of the pattern of forced and bored listening. We want to change this whole dynamic, and it isn't just up to the speakers to change and connect to the listener. The feminine must also rise up and shift what's happening so that listening is exciting and creates union as well.

Listeners as "Takers"

This is when people ask us questions that we don't want to answer. Someone wants us to fill their bowl. This might be where someone goes up to a famous person and asks, "Hey, what are you doing?" and keeps asking them questions as the famous person tries to take a quiet stroll alone. Or it's being cornered by a relative at a

Christmas party and they're asking you a bunch of personal questions that you don't want to answer because it is none of their business.

This is similar to the "takers" that we talked about previously. They want you to talk (masculine) so that they can receive (feminine). But because they are asking for things you don't want to give, they are actually taking, which has nothing to do with union or connection.

When in the presence of these kinds of takers, it's important to know that we are under no obligation to answer questions if we don't want to. They are asking us to give them something that we don't want to give. It would be the same as if someone asked you to give them $1000. You wouldn't feel obligated to give it to them. In the same way, we don't have to answer a question just because it was asked.

Teachers & Students

In School

> *"It is the supreme art of the teacher*
> *to awaken joy in creative expression and knowledge."*
> ALBERT EINSTEIN

In many situations, children are forced to attend school. They have no choice. The teacher is simply showing up for work as well. If there is a connection between the teacher and students, the students will share what they need with the teacher. The teacher will then be happy to give it. These are the happy moments in school that we remember for many years to come.

However, if there is no connection between the students and the teacher, then the teacher simply presents the work. The students pretend to listen and retain very little. These are the horrible (and most common) days that we remember from school.

Regular school is a classic example of the masculine being forced upon the feminine. The nature of the feminine is irrelevant. This is in no way meant to disrespect people who choose to be teachers. Many teachers go into the profession because of a desire to truly teach and help children learn (including both of my parents). However, this is not how many school programs are designed, and the teachers end up with their hands tied.

Tabula Rasa

In most mainstream schools in the West, a curriculum is given to the teachers to present to the students. The students are graded from 0 to 100 based on their ability to understand and repeat the curriculum back on tests. If a child gets 50%, it is their responsibility to try to understand or take in more of what was given. The onus is seldom on the teacher to change how they are teaching so that the child can receive 100% of what is being taught.

Can you see how this is backward? The student (feminine) is simply judged and counted. They are not treated as a sentient, whole being. This is based on the theory that children's minds are *tabula rasa*, or "clear slates." Their minds are simply there to be filled, and some children will be able to take in more than others.

This also speaks to the idea that the feminine is simply the absence of the masculine. The feminine has no real essence of its own. The masculine must simply fill it without regarding the already present wisdom and desires of the feminine. The feminine is just a board to be written upon.

As previously mentioned, children must sit and listen whether they are interested or not. If they are not interested and are not able to fake it, they are considered "problem children," or they may even have some kind of "attention disorder." Can you imagine being told that you have an attention disorder because you don't want to listen to something you aren't interested in?

This begins as soon as we are socialized, and because we are so young, we don't even know that it's happening. All we know is that there is someone at the front of the class to whom we have to listen, or else we'll be punished. Our only job is to listen, sit still, and "be good."

And yet, there are brilliant teachers out there. If we're lucky, we can all remember at least one teacher who was truly connected to their students. They taught what the students wanted to learn, and union happened. That teacher who you connected with became your favourite teacher for life.

SPIRITUAL TEACHERS

Imagine that you find a teacher or guru from whom you truly want to learn. You sign up for a class with them. As you sit there eagerly awaiting what they are going to share, the teacher will feel this feminine receptivity. When this receptivity is felt, a true teacher will respond to the group and teach whatever it is that the students are looking to learn. It might even mean teaching something very different than what was planned, which, of course, is perfect.

In this state, masculine and feminine are joined. The masculine feeds the feminine what is desired. The feminine opens up her heart, and this vacuum draws wisdom from the Divine through the Teacher. We experience incredible bliss here—true, incredible, heart-opening bliss. It is in this union that transmission can happen. When both the teacher's and student's hearts are open, much more will be passed from masculine to feminine than just the words spoken.

Teachers vs Presenters

A teacher speaks in response to the needs of their students. This is why when you watch talks by gurus of the past, there is a moment when they look around the room and just seem to be breathing and observing. Then, they simply start talking, speaking directly to those present in the room.

Alternatively, presenters already have what they are going to say before they start speaking. It doesn't matter who's in the room.

They will give the same talk over and over again. This can work when we are teaching something like accounting or some kind of process that doesn't change based on who's participating. It also works if someone is presenting an academic idea to see who will grasp it or not. The goal here isn't union with the group. It is simply to present a topic, and maybe there will be a question-and-answer period later where more connection is possible.

When we are learning topics that are more expansive, like spirituality, having a true teacher is a wonderful blessing because we will learn exactly what we need to hear at that moment. Every individual journey needs different things at each point, so a canned speech that is repeatable regardless of the audience simply doesn't fit.

Reading the Room

When I began doing talks about my books and teaching spiritual studies, I was nervous because I am quite shy in large groups. However, years ago, my teacher told me to stop rehearsing everything I was going to say in my head. He said that I could simply trust that the right words would come.

So, when I started speaking in front of groups, I would prepare a sketch of what I wanted to say to make sure I made the point that I wanted to share. Then, I would get up on stage, take a deep breath, and simply trust whatever came to me.

I often found myself telling random stories that didn't seem to go together. I even found myself turning my head from one side of the room to the other as I changed channels and started a new story. After a while, there would be a moment when the energy of the room would change. You could hear a pin drop. The whole room was completely in tune, and it was as if I was only speaking to one person. That's when the actual talk would begin. I would speak, and the room would be absolutely silent. It was so magical.

Afterwards, people would come up to me and say, "How did you know to tell that story? That was just what I needed to hear. It was as if you were speaking directly to me."

My sense of what happens is that, in the beginning, everyone has their own personal questions and it is as if I "hear" them and answer them. Once everyone's questions are answered, it is like the group is then sewn into a whole. There is a beautiful union, and it is very memorable.

Performers & Audiences

There is something magical about watching a performer connect with their audience. The very presence of the audience lights them up. When the audience is animated and enthralled, the performer performs in ways they have never experienced. They sing differently. The energy in the room is alive, and the music is amazing because the energy of the audience moves the performer.

It is a completely different experience when the performer is off in their own world. The audience will go off into their own world as well. Or maybe you are playing in a bar and the audience is off in their own world. You have no one to play for, and there is no union with the audience possible there either.

If we have been hired to play background music or to create ambience, then we must find our bliss in the union of ourselves and our instrument. This can be a beautiful union. You can play what you're inspired to play. You can feel one with yourself and the music. The audience and the event just become an opportunity to play in the mojo of other people without the goal of connecting with them.

Meeting Your Audience

I have a friend who is a spiritual singer. She sings songs of goddesses, light, and healing. One day, she was telling me how frustrating it was to sing for some groups in Canada. It was like they weren't even there, she couldn't connect with them, and it was hard for her to find joy in it. However, when she sang for groups in India, it was like the audience was a part of her. She wanted that experience here but didn't know how to make it happen or what she was doing wrong.

The difference was that in India, she offered what that audience desired. They were spiritual communities seeking an exalted experience. All the music that came through her perfectly matched their feminine desire. However, back home in Canada, she would often perform for local groups and events that weren't so devout in their spiritual journeys or who weren't spiritual at all. She would still perform at the events because her music was healing, and maybe there was someone there who would really get it.

However, the audience wasn't seeking it. No matter how beautiful a gift she had to give them, it wouldn't seem beautiful to an unreceptive audience. It would be like performing classical music to an audience who wanted to hear hard rock. Whether your music is beautiful or not is irrelevant. If it isn't what the audience desires, there can be no union… unless you happen to have some hard rock up your sleeve.

Your Personal Journey:

Strengthening the Feminine

1. Do you enjoy listening to other people? Who do you know that really speaks to you about things you are interested in? Are there others who talk regardless of who is listening?
2. If the speaker is off in their own world, are you able to shift a conversation to something of interest to both of you?
3. Have you had great teachers in your life with whom you easily relax into the student role? Who are they?
4. Have you had the experience of being in an audience where the performers and the audience are completely connected?

Strengthening the Masculine

1. Are you careful to speak about things your listener is interested in?

2. Are you good at explaining things in a language that everyone can understand?
3. Do you enjoy being in the role of teacher? This could be in a job, at work, with family, or anywhere that you are sharing something to help others.
4. Who are great role models for you who spoke in ways that created union with themselves and others?

MASCULINE & FEMININE DYNAMICS

Chapter 6

Structure & Chaos

Writing this book was a fascinating journey between Structure and Chaos.

It began years ago with observing the chaotic world of relationships. Why did some work and others didn't? What were all the control issues about? Why does the spark go out? What's the difference between that happy couple and this frustrated one? There seemed to be no particular pattern that made sense (chaos).

And then patterns started to form (structure and order). There was the yin/yang dynamic from Chinese philosophies. There was the dance of the masculine and feminine energies in Tantra. There was the difference between what happened in loving connection with another, and what happened in separation and the need to overpower others. A structure was beginning to form that made sense of this wild world of love and relationships and perhaps could help us to navigate it.

My studies intensified. I began to teach courses and give live talks about the masculine and feminine. Once I became single, it became the foundation of my dating experience. I even wrote the book Tales of the Tinderverse recounting my journey in the world of online dating seeking a truly masculine partner.

Eventually, it was time to bring all of these teachings and experiences together into the book you are holding right now. It began as pure chaos. I gathered transcriptions of all the talks and courses I had given, notes from my studies, and memories from my life. It was a chaotic hodgepodge of over 104,000 words. Structure (my editor) entered the scene and said this was far too much. The editing team did a structural edit of the manuscript and handed it back to me to sort out.

MASCULINE & FEMININE DYNAMICS

As I swam through their critiques, I couldn't find the proper flow. So, I meditated. I sat still (structure) and listened for answers. I left the manuscript alone for a while to clear my head and then picked it up again as inspiration came (chaos). The aha moment came and I was able to reorganize the book so that I could explore each topic as was needed. The editing team completed the line edits and proof. Phew. I figured that it was time to publish! Perfect!

Alas, something inside of me was said, "Not yet". This is also chaos because it wasn't part of the structure I had planned. It was unexpected. In this chaos, my intuition was guiding me to slow down and wait. So, my masculine desire to continue supported that and took his foot off of the gas.

After a couple of weeks, I had the inspiration to start recording the audio version. As I sat down in the recording studio and started to read out loud, I realized that the book wasn't flowing properly in my voice. The solid container of the recording process created a clear space for me to realize that what I had written wasn't quite right. My true creativity and wisdom (chaos) weren't actually being shared.

I was so disappointed. I had become attached to my publishing date (structure). I wanted to force the book out (oppress chaos), but I couldn't. So, I waited.

A few days later, I had a conversation with a woman who was struggling to connect with her feminine side. She had been in the army and was completely self-sufficient. Being vulnerable and open in relationships was a challenge, but that's what she wanted. I asked her if she wanted to read my manuscript. Maybe it would help. I told her that it was basically finished, but if she saw anything amok, I'd appreciate her feedback. The next time I looked at my manuscript (the online version I had shared with her), it was covered in corrections and places where she was confused. This was essential feedback as she had been a student of mine for years. She had heard many of my talks about the masculine and feminine. If she was confused about what I was saying, then I definitely had to explain things better.

At this point, another friend of mine popped into my head. She'd been involved in the creation of many of my previous books and knew me very well. When she called me the next day, rather synchronistically, I asked if

STRUCTURE & CHAOS

she would also take a look at my manuscript. Perhaps I needed more critical eyes on it. She happily agreed to take a look.

Alas, so many more edits were needed. She knew me and my teachings well, and felt that I was holding back and not putting it all out there. I wasn't going into the deep stuff that she knew was part of my romantic and day-to-day experiences.

This was not what I was expecting. I love deadlines. I love masculine structure. I love sticking to a plan. She was asking me to re-vision huge parts of the book and take the time to dive deeper within myself to see what I was leaving out. I could feel my masculine structure wanting to put the brakes on – to say "No. The book is fine. Just let it go!"

But I couldn't. If there is anything I've learned in my life is that there is great wisdom in the chaos. There is great wisdom when things aren't lining up according to plan. This is where something really new and amazing will be created.

So, my masculine structure chose to embrace the chaos and slowly stepped through all of my friends' corrections, points of confusion, and suggestions. My masculine breathed deeply in order to maintain our forward direction as I came across each new thought. I released the stress of the deadlines that my masculine had tried to impose and allowed the creative process to flow.

Eventually, the chaotic birth process was complete. My masculine had come through being fully supportive at every step… and a new life was born.

The challenge is that we have mostly experienced the controlling version of structure—within ourselves, within relationships, and within the world. Because we have been taught to be uncomfortable with the unknown, chaos, and wildness, we have liked how structure and order are used to control and oppress chaos and mystery.

Because of this, structure and order (masculine) have become the only side of this dynamic that we desire. Any sense of mystery and chaos (feminine) has been feared, misunderstood, and totally avoided. We have been taught to have a stiff upper lip instead of allowing emotions to flow. We create false security by telling ourselves that what is tangible is all that is real. We make sure people do well in science and math and ignore children's passion for the arts. We try to tame our partners so that they are predictable, so that we feel safer. We try to control our children by moulding them into who we want them to be instead of trusting the mystery of who they might become.

The answer is understanding the exciting union of structure and chaos. We want to look at how structure supports creation from chaos. We want to see how new things are manifested through trusting that something new and unknown is possible.

What is Structure?

Structure and order are used interchangeably as the masculine side of this dynamic. They are all about creating the conditions for creation to happen. They are about supporting feminine chaos and wildness. Everything is created out of the feminine. This is where new ideas come from. This is where the colour of life is. This is where creation comes from.

Let's say you have a new idea (feminine). The masculine within you then comes in to create the plan to make it happen. If you have inspiration for a song, the masculine grabs the guitar and starts playing. As our emotions respond to the world around us, our inner masculine is the stillness within where we can unpack what our emotions are telling us.

Structure is the spreadsheets that transform a dream into a business plan. Parenting creates a supportive structure that allows children to expand and grow into who they are. Structure is facilitating a workshop so that others can have a deep and meaningful experience.

What are some ways that we can create structure for those around us?

Healthy Work Environments

A strong structure in the workplace allows for incredible creativity from the staff. This structure could be reliable management policies. It could be transparency when it comes to pay raises and schedules. It can also be the security for an employee to know that they will have a job tomorrow. They know that the owners and management have everything in order. They know that they can just relax and focus on their job without worry.

If there are creative endeavours, then the structure could be a brainstorming session where everyone gathers in a room and states the question. Then, the facilitators ask the room for any and all ideas to come forward. This is the time for chaos and crazy ideas. This is where we stimulate our creativity and come up with new things we have never tried before. The key to success here is that there are no bad ideas in this phase. We trust the process of chaos and enjoy where the wildness takes us. After all the ideas are out on the table, structure can come back in and start to see which ones could fit into a new plan.

Holding Space for Others

This is where we provide stillness for another person's chaos.

Sometimes we are so upset, the chaos and uncertainty are overwhelming. We could be angry, grieving, sad, or simply emotionally overwhelmed by something. This is a very chaotic state. We can't find the straight way through.

Ideally, our inner masculine will help us to slow down, breathe, and be still enough to feel whatever is going on. Our masculine may pick up a journal to write out what's happening. We may grab pillows and pound our fists into them or go for a run to help release the emotions. These are all ways that our own masculine can support our feminine experience.

However, there are times when our inner masculine isn't big enough to handle the immensity of the emotions we are dealing with. Maybe it's a new experience that we can't fathom. Maybe it's a sadness or grief that completely overwhelms us. Or maybe it's a fury that we aren't sure we can handle without doing something rash that we will regret later.

This is why it's important to have people in our lives who can be that strong masculine for us. It is easier for them to hold stillness for us because their mind hasn't been taken offline by their emotions. We just need to know that this friend will polarize all the way to the masculine side so that we can dive deep. It's like scuba diving. The more we trust the person on the boat holding the rope, the deeper we can go.

This is where we can call a friend who will provide masculine strength and stillness for us. Together, we will create a new whole where their masculine structural state will balance our feminine chaotic state.

The goal of this interaction is to get to the core of our emotions because there is always a truth hiding in there that is important to get to.

The key to holding space for another is to stay in sober stillness. We are the shoulder to cry on. We might say a couple of things here and there, but it is not about fixing the other person. We are there to support their feminine journey into chaos. It is not about rescuing them by pulling them up too soon. We want them to be able to dive deeply into the struggle, with faith that they are held in the sacred process of this union.

We also don't dive into the chaos with them. We don't tell them our own stories so they know we understand. We don't add to the emotions or the drama. We have polarized in the other direction so that we can support their dive. We are still. We are strength. We are the person on the boat holding the line as they dive deep. They know that no matter how deep they go, we'll pull them out if they give us the right tug. This is the strength of friendship and love.

STRUCTURE & CHAOS

This masculine-feminine dynamic has nothing to do with gender or polarity preference. Even if you prefer the masculine role in relationships, it is not your job to always hold space for your feminine partner. This dynamic is based on each situation because there are times when we all need to dive deeply into our own chaos and emotions. We all lose loved ones and feel grief. We all get confused and could use a sounding board. We all feel hurt, sad, and lost at times.

This is where we all need to be able to connect with our own feminine to create balance within.

Artistic Benefactors

Sometimes, we hear of artists or musicians living with others who want to support their craft. They may offer to give them a place to live and whatever materials they need so that the artist can just focus on their art. These benefactors (masculine) create a beautiful union with the creative artist (feminine). It is a win/win because the artist has the freedom to dive into their chaos and mystery, and the benefactor gets to support and enjoy what is created. This often happened with inventors as well. Inventors like Nikola Tesla often needed a financier (masculine) to give him the freedom to dive completely into the inspired and creative (feminine) aspects of his experiments.

The key is that when an artist or an inventor has a benefactor creating structure, the benefactor does not tell them what they are allowed to create. This would be control. Instead, the benefactor says to the artist, "Here's a studio. Here are the canvases. Here's the clay. Here's everything you need. Please create. I have so much faith in you." The artist is totally free in this beautiful union. They can go right to the edge of their chaos—to the edge of their creative capacity.

It begins with love, connection, honour, and trust. The masculine loves creating the structure because they want to see what the feminine is going to create. In the same way, the feminine is incredibly grateful and appreciative of the masculine for what they give. They think, "How blessed am I that I have this incredible support and structure to play within? Amazing!"

And from that incredible support and gratitude, amazing and new things are born.

Structure in Parenting

> *"Before I got married,*
> *I had six theories about raising children;*
> *Now, I have six children and no theories."*
> JOHN WILMOT

Being a parent is a masculine role because children are always in the feminine. They receive what they need from us. They are growing in beautiful chaos. We protect them because they are vulnerable. Who they are is unknown—even to them. Our primary role as a parent is to be the masculine structure for them to grow into whatever they are meant to become. It is about creating security so that they can explore the wild mystery that they are. If we can create a safe home where they always know there's food, love, and support, they can truly grow and thrive.

Although structure isn't about being controlling, we can still have rules within a family home to create safety for everyone. I have two children (currently in their 20s). When they were teenagers, we had a rule that no one should ever have to worry. If they were out late, they just had to call and update us as to where they were. It wasn't a strict curfew. It was just a simple structure that we could allow for the chaotic experiences of teenagers.

When children are small, the structure might be a dependable bedtime routine, breakfast before school, etc. It might be that you couldn't be mean to your siblings or have a snack within a certain time before meals. All of these small things create an external structure that they can depend on. And because they don't have to worry about these things, they can focus on being a kid.

For some, this structure wasn't there growing up. I had one friend whose mom struggled financially. So, if my friend wanted to have a home phone (there were only landlines then), she had to work and pay for it from age fifteen until she moved out. Other friends had parents with addiction issues or who struggled with depression. There was no structure or safety in the home, and the kids responded in many different ways.

Sometimes, they rose up and became the masculine structure that their parents weren't. They cleaned up after them. They paid the utility bills. They cooked and did anything needed to create balance in the home. Those children lost their childhood. It was the end of the chaotic, mysterious growth of that seed. They will often be stunted at that point in their childhood because they had to become an adult early. I'm not saying they can't heal this and recover their innocence. They may just spend a lot of time with counsellors and healers on the journey to get there.

Sometimes, the child continued down that chaotic path themselves and never experienced what it is to have structure. They end up not trusting structure of any kind. They fight against authority and don't want any rules. They simply continue that unbalanced life that they grew up with. It is not evil, wrong, or a sign of poor character. It is just all they have ever known.

Then there is the opposite situation where the parents are over-controlling. Control is not structure. The intention of control is to minimize chaos and the unknown as opposed to honouring and dancing with them. Sometimes, this is done with the hope of being good parents, wanting to do the right thing for their children. So, they create as much structure and security as possible. Perhaps the control comes out of fear because we had a hard time growing up and saw too much, and we don't want that for our children. Maybe we personally are afraid of the world and just want to keep our children safe. Sometimes, we are controlling in all of our relationships and are no different with our children.

However, control limits the true growth of the child. Growth, by nature, is chaotic. Chaos is not a bad thing. It is simply all that is uncharted and unstructured. Each of our true paths is chaotic by nature. We are each unique individuals, and as parents, control can easily stifle that natural organic growth that allows children to grow into who they truly are.

This control can look like many things. It can be telling our kids who they can or can't hang out with, what classes they must take at school, that they have to play hockey, or what to wear. It can also be over-planning their lives. We may have ideas about what we want our children to accomplish so we plan, plan, and plan some more. Between all of our plans and their schoolwork, children can easily end up with no downtime. No room for organic growth or thought. Everything has already been decided.

Sometimes, the children rebel, and they become the absolute opposite. To the same extent that their parents were out of balance by being controlling, they go to the imbalanced, chaotic side. They never want any structure, and they don't want anyone to tell them what to do.

Perhaps they will go along with their parents' vision for them, and their mysterious and chaotic growth pattern ends. They simply fall into step with the plan. Sometimes it works out. Sometimes it doesn't. If it doesn't, at some point in their adulthood, they will have to destroy almost everything (normally unconsciously) back to the point where they gave in to their parents' plan so that they can start growing anew according to their true soul's path.

What is Feminine Chaos?

"The only constant in life is change."
HERACLITUS

Chaos is not crazy destruction and insanity. Chaos is mystery, unknown, flow, and deep emotional truth. Chaos holds all the possibilities of creation. It is not a negative thing or something to be avoided.

Yet we have been taught to fear chaos because we are uncomfortable with the unknown. We have succumbed to the belief that we can control the Universe with our intellect and the understanding of things. But after being alive for a certain number of years, we soon realize that chaos is the foundation of life. We truly never know what is going to happen.

Chaos is the birth of all things. To swim in chaos is to happily release all attachments and trust in the Universe. It is trusting that all things grow, change, die, and are reborn. Chaos allows the cycle of life, which is what leads to new ideas being created.

Let's look at an example of structure that minimizes chaos vs structure that helps us explore chaos.

We could set up play areas inside a school where children would play with one toy for ten minutes and then move on to the next one. Each child must be in each station for exactly 10 minutes. This would be excellent if the goal was to teach the children a very specific skill. Each area would allow them to practise something until they had everything down pat. This is not about creativity or individual expression. A specific skill is being taught. Very little chaos or creativity at all.

However, if we put those children into the woods and let them play, chaos is possible. The structure is organizing the bus to get there and chaperones to ensure everyone's safety. Within this container, the children get to access their creativity. They get to be spontaneous and respond to whatever happens. There is no goal except for the exploration of the unknown within each child.

In chaos, brand-new things can be born. If you observe these children in the woods, very interesting things will happen because we aren't controlling the possibilities. Each child will make different and unexpected choices. They will interact here and there, and brand new and interesting things will happen.

Chaos is where the vision of an artist comes from—not from figures on a spreadsheet. Spreadsheets can be useful in the manifestation process for sure. We are not negating the importance of the masculine balance here, but the feminine is the inspiration to create the spreadsheet in the first place.

MASCULINE & FEMININE DYNAMICS

We have been taught that chaos is to be avoided and that not knowing what's going to happen next is scary. Some of this certainly comes from our history. If we have experienced war, famine, or economic depression, chaos can be very scary. It can mean death, loss, or not feeding your family. The desire for security, the desire for structure, the desire for the comfort of knowing what's going to happen tomorrow is also very natural.

The problem comes when we no longer want to see chaos, mystery, or the unknown. If we push it aside as if it isn't real or is to be shunned, life becomes very boring. And worse, we lose our ability to navigate chaos. We only know how to follow prescribed rules and systems.

However, the real world isn't made of rules and systems. The world is based in chaos. So, we end up not being able to navigate the real world at all.

Blackfoot Wisdom

In many Native belief systems, it is understood that the world is made of spirit, and spirit is chaotic by nature. This leads to realizing that we are living in a constant state of flux—from energy to matter and back again. Chaos is simply the unmanifested building blocks of life.

Knowing this allows them to live in a constant state of renewal—always shifting and changing. Spirit and chaos are completely honoured in that cycle of life.

From here, other aspects of their lives are based on this reality. They realize that each person must learn to be intuitive. How else could you navigate? Whereas the Western mind want us to believe that science can map the world and even control it. This gives us a feeling of safety, even though every day, we see that life is not so simple—not the weather, our health, or the actions of people.

A wise woman once told me, "Darling, the world isn't black and white—this is only a belief of the young. Once you've lived as long as I have," (she was in her 70s), "you'll realize that the world is mostly gray."

Change is the only constant.

Embracing the Wild Feminine

Sometimes, we fear wildness, to be feral and untamed. If I am wild, am I just crazy? Am I out of control? Well, yes. But it's not what you think.

How do wild horses act in nature? Are they running helter-skelter all over the place and acting crazy? No, of course not. They are just living the natural life of a horse. They are eating food, having babies, and sleeping. They move when there is danger and rest when it is safe. They live according to their instinct. They are connected within and to their environment.

Are they out of control? Yes, they are not controlled.

If humans want to use the horse in some way, we now want to control it. We want to remove this wildness. We want to "tame" the horse so that we can feel safe. We need to know that we are in control and that the horse has no say. It must act as an object that only does what we tell it to. Otherwise, we don't feel safe. If the horse doesn't like what we are doing to it, it will naturally attack us and could harm or kill us. So, we do whatever it takes to make sure that the horse is tamed—under control—and there is no wildness left.

The same thing has happened to us. We have been tamed. Our wildness didn't fit into our family homes. It definitely didn't fit into our school systems. We had to be forced to do whatever it took to oppress any wildness within us, and if it snuck out, we were punished or labeled as difficult and "out of control."

In the tantric belief system, this wildness is very important. This is our connection to our truth, our reality, and who we truly are. To truly understand a horse, we would have to observe it in its natural

MASCULINE & FEMININE DYNAMICS

habitat. It is the same with us. To observe ourselves tamed and in captivity is not a true vision of what it is to be human any more than we can understand horses based on one tied up in a stable.

Tantra assumes that we all have great wisdom within us and that we are perfectly formed beings. All external, controlling structures cut us off from our deepest wisdom. To be tantric means that we are fully alive and trust the wisdom in our wildness. We know that anything can happen at any moment. This is the excitement of what it feels like to be alive!

So, how do we bring back our wildness? The first step is to trust it — to trust the feminine within. We need to trust that if there were no rules, and we were wild, untamed, and uncivilized, we would still be who we are. It is a curious belief to think that we make choices only based on the rules that are being imposed on us because the truth is, we often will find a way to do what we desire regardless of the rules.

Einstein once said that the most important question we have to ask ourselves is if we believe the world is a safe place. My interpretation of that, especially in this context, is that if I trust that the world is a safe place, then it will be easier to trust my wildness, my intuition, and my deep feminine. I will trust that if I listen, and act on my inner guidance, things will turn out just fine.

If I don't believe that the world is a safe place, then we must explore what it means to be wild. What if trusting our wild senses will keep us alive? What if our wildness taps into a reality that is deeper and older than the world that makes us feel so unsafe? Our journey then becomes to trust our primal self and "wild" senses — allowing our wild feminine to lead the charge, and our strong masculine to take the necessary steps to lead us on a path of safety.

Trusting Mystery & the Unknown

"Mystery creates wonder and wonder is the basis of man's desire to understand."
NEIL ARMSTRONG

Mystery is another aspect of feminine chaos that has been put on the back burner or deleted altogether. Our world likes to focus on what we can see, touch, taste, feel, smell, or hear. We trust what we can see, count, and understand. This is the masculine.

The feminine is the unseen. The feminine is everything that we can't experience with our five senses. This is when you know something inside, and others say, "How do you know that? You can't prove it." Yet you know it anyway.

This is terrifying to many people. There is a reason that people were burned at the stake and called witches because they shouldn't have known what they knew. Those desiring power cannot control the unseen, and therefore, we are taught to never trust it.

Yet mystery is what makes life exciting. Mystery is everything that is coming. It is all of the unknown within us. It is what we do not yet know about our romantic partners. It is wondering who our children will grow into being. It is wondering what today will bring.

If we live as if there is no mystery, life becomes very boring, and we miss the potential of many situations. If we assume that we know everything there is to know about our partners, then we stop asking them questions and diving deeper into them. If we already have an idea of who our children should be and don't allow their unique mysteries to unfold, they will either distance themselves from us so their soul can express its true path, or they will live within our ideas, a fraction of who they really are.

If we don't allow mystery into our days, we will walk through them like a robot. Whether we are working or retired, we will expect today to be much like yesterday. Even if new ideas pop in, we probably can't fit them into our schedules. If unexpected things happen, we may complain about them instead of embracing that something new and different is occurring!

One of my favourite movies about living this way is Moana. It is a Disney animated movie about being an adventurer in life, going out into the world, and not knowing what you are going to find. This is a very different experience than knowing what you want, going out, and finding it. Instead, we trust that there are things in the world that we don't know, but we still want to go and find them. This requires a whole different adventurous mechanism inside. It is a completely different muscle that allows us to go out and trust that there are things to discover that we don't know.

It is exciting to swim in that mystery. We get to trust that we can do it. All we have to do is trust ourselves that we are strong enough to meet any challenge no matter what comes our way. Very, very exciting!

"I Don't Know"

> *"There are more things in heaven and earth, Horatio, than are dreamt of in your philosophy."*
> WILLIAM SHAKESPEARE, HAMLET

One of the most powerful sayings that help us honour the mystery of life is, "I don't know." When someone says, "Why did that happen?", some part of us wants to create an answer, but it won't be true. Because the truth is that we don't know.

Why did their marriage split up? I don't know. We might try to list all the things we can see, but we don't really know. Why did I have to be born to those parents? I don't know. Why don't I want to go to the party? I don't know. Why don't I want to have children? I don't know.

Because we are comfortable in the masculine "known" world, we will try to give an answer. Their marriage split up because they didn't love each other anymore, he went bankrupt, she hated his parents, or she had an affair. We will grasp any bit of information

STRUCTURE & CHAOS

we have and try to come up with a reason. However, the world is made of mystery. Maybe it was karmic patterns they were living out. Maybe they were meant to meet someone else. Maybe, maybe, maybe.

In the end, we really don't know.

There are things in this world that we can understand. A car, for example, was made by humans. We can understand everything about the inner workings of a car because they are limited and we understand the purpose of every part. However, we can't understand what goes on within a human body, mind, or spirit. We didn't create it. We can try to map it, make names for all the parts, and observe how they seem to interact, but there are entire other processes going on that we don't understand.

How do emotions affect our bodies? How does our spiritual connection affect our health? How do hurricanes happen? How does the solar system work? Maybe there is no time-space continuum. Maybe it is just a fabrication in our minds. Maybe we are all really in one spot, in total bliss right now. Maybe it is all an illusion. We can never know.

The goal is to enjoy the balance between the known and the unknown. There are things we can know and that's important. It is great to drive cars, speak Spanish, make amazing French toast, and balance a chequebook. These experiences are all brilliant.

Then, we can also love everything we don't know and honour the mystery that life is. This is where we start to see miracles and amazing things happen. However, when we don't allow for mystery, we create a very small box for an infinite experience, and when we only live within the box, we run the risk of only seeing what's inside of it.

But what if the box isn't actually real? What if it is just something we have created because we have been taught to not trust the unknown and mystery in life? When we remove this box, we get to learn to honour mystery and walk through life saying, "I have no idea why I'm doing this, but it will be an adventure. Let's see what happens!"

Allowing Emotions to Flow

Very often, our chaos and wildness began to be oppressed in our childhood. Let's say that you were crying, upset, or freaking out. How often did our parents say, "Alright. Let's sit on the couch and talk. I'm here for you. What's going on?"

Instead, most kids are told to go to their rooms until they can "be civil" or until they are "feeling better." This sends a very clear message that it's not okay to be upset. It's not okay to be messy. It's not okay to be "out of control."

The first time I went to a tantra retreat in California, we were doing all kinds of exercises to try to trigger our buried emotions. All kinds of traumas and issues in our current or past relationships came up. Because it was an emotionally safe place to dive into these buried struggles, there was often a lot of intense feeling, yelling, and crying.

Afterwards, we would sit in a circle and discuss what was coming up for us. On the first day, one of the leaders said, "If someone starts to cry, do not offer them a tissue. If they specifically ask for one, that's okay, but don't offer it to them."

When we offer a tissue to someone who is crying, we are sending a message saying, "Clean yourself up. You don't want to be like that." Instead, if you just let someone cry with tears and snot flowing down their face, we send them a clear message that it is okay to be messy. Maybe they need to feel externally the same messiness that they feel on the inside. It is okay to have a wide range of emotions. It is okay to have a messy life. It is okay to dive into that chaos. It is all part of a whole life.

However, we are not taught how to allow people to do that. Imagine being with someone and them just honouring your emotions—truly being seen. There is something so powerful about someone else looking right into your eyes and saying, "Go for it.

Your feelings matter. What you're going through right now is real, and it is important. I'm listening." As opposed to someone who says, "Hey, everyone has something going on. We've all been there. It's not that big a deal. Let's do something to take your mind off of this."

For a lot of us, that has been our experience. It has been our experience at work, with our parents, at school, with our friends, with our partners, and even with our children. Then, we internalize their response which becomes the voice of our inner masculine. Before long, when an emotion comes up, our inner voice is chastising us saying, "Well, that's not a reasonable feeling. That's ridiculous. That's not enlightened. That is not calm and mature! Get over yourself." Our inner voice can be quite brutal.

After many years of listening to this inner voice chastise us for having feelings, we easily allow others to chastise us as well. We are familiar with it. We unconsciously expect them to treat us the same way that we treat ourselves.

However, our masculine structure should always strengthen, support, and expand our feminine chaos. This is what allows us to heal the deepest parts of ourselves. This is what allows us to manifest our wildest and craziest desires. This is when we truly feel alive!

Plan & Spontaneity

"Let planning be the springboard,
so that spontaneity can be our splash."
ROBIN SHARMA

A practical example of this dynamic is plan and spontaneity. Let's say you are going on a trip. Maybe you want to plan (masculine) every single detail—where you are going to be, how long you are going to spend at each place, where you are going to stay, how you are going to get there, etc. Yet, other people just want to go by the seat of their pants (feminine). Neither one is wrong, but we have a much more enjoyable experience if we allow both to dance together.

If we only want the masculine plan, it will be hard when things don't happen as we expected because we will be attached to everything playing out as planned. It's important to have some spontaneous spirit to allow for planes to be delayed, for that "perfect" restaurant that we wanted to go to not to be open, or for something better to happen that we couldn't have known ahead of time was possible. When we allow spontaneity, chaos, and mystery into our plans, our experiences become very rich, and our ability to flow allows for great peace inside.

On the flip side, let's say that you want to be 100% spontaneous and have no plan at all. This can be quite stressful if you haven't booked a place to stay, and don't know when your flights are. It is nice to know that you have enough money in your pocket to pay for a nice dinner or to go on that amazing excursion. We can still be carefree and trust that the perfect opportunity will arise. The key is that the masculine serves the feminine. So, while we are being spontaneous and inspired, we simply ask our masculine to make the plans to support our amazing adventure.

Structure & Chaos Within

> *"One must still have chaos in oneself to be able to give birth to a dancing star."*
> NIETZCHE

When we bring this dynamic dance within, we feel free to be who we truly are. This is where our inner masculine fully supports our wildness, our uniqueness, and our current response to the world around us. This is where we feel completely alive because our masculine rises up and creates whatever structure and safety we need to experience whatever we feel at that moment.

Osho used to talk about becoming "Zorba the Buddha." His idea was that we should live life to the fullest like "Zorba the Greek" with the inner stillness and presence of the Buddha.

Can you imagine the fullness of life when we can be all of these things? To be like the Buddha — still, listening, receptive, quiet, and deep — and then to also have the wildness, unpredictability, freedom, and excitement of Zorba — never knowing what's coming next, but knowing that you will be able to respond perfectly from your deepest centre.

This is where we find our personal balance and inner joy.

Most of us tend toward either chaos or order. If we are very left-brained, we will tend toward order all of the time. If we are more right-brained, we will prefer the freedom to "stay in the flow", not wanting the restrictions of discipline and order.

But we need both. Once we know that there is food on the table and the bills are paid, we can have all the freedom in the world to expand, create, and do whatever we want. This is what creates the dynamic balance of peace and excitement in our lives.

Chaos & Mystery Within

"Mystery is what makes a woman, woman.
A woman without mystery is no woman.
She is a girl who has yet discovered the depths of her heart."

The above quote can apply to the feminine within all genders. This is that point in our lives when we begin to trust and plumb our own mystery. This is when we stop imagining that we know everything there is to know within us. As the quote above says, it is an interesting time of maturity.

The feminine within is the part of us that we cannot know and cannot control. It is truly our wild nature. In many societies, it is neither honoured nor explored. Instead, it is often broken out of us. Sometimes people are born into families of artists, and it is very much nurtured, but that is generally not the norm.

Let's imagine that at this moment, you actually don't know who you are — that there is a wildness and mystery within that has never been tapped. Perhaps you wouldn't know what you do with it, you have been afraid, or you don't know what you'd find. It is partly this fear of mystery that causes us to hide so much of our true nature deep in our subconscious.

As our subconscious becomes filled with everything that we are afraid of about ourselves, we develop more and more "triggers" in life. As we walk through our days, we are suddenly angry about something, suddenly sad, or we have unrequited hopes and dreams that we don't believe will ever happen. They all live in this unknown, chaotic, and mysterious place, and we don't know what would happen if we started to look at them. So, we just say, "I'm not going to think about it, I am going to go back to logic and structure. It's safer there."

Emotional Chaos

When we understand that chaos isn't a negative thing, that it is simply unstructured and uncontrolled, we can see how our emotions are by definition chaotic. They are our responses to the outside world. Because we are multidimensional, multi-layered, and unique individuals, it is only reasonable that our natural responses to things will be unique and not according to any external structure.

This is why our emotions are so valuable. This is why they have so much to share. In a world that tends to value logic and structure above all things, our emotional response says, "Yes, I can see that you would like me to respond in that way, but that simply isn't my Truth. This is my Truth."

This is why we end up with a lot of buried fury — anger that has been suppressed for a long time. Healthy anger tells us that what is currently going on is not okay. Yet as children, this opinion was seldom important, heard, or cared about. In fact, if there was abuse in the home, the only thing you could do was bury your anger, your masculine protector, because it would only get worse if you didn't.

If you find yourself having outbursts of anger and rage, this is an indicator that there is something buried deep within that is ready to be looked at. It's an important clue to the beginning of the breadcrumb trail that, once uncovered and resolved, will bring a brand new inner peace.

Many people have a lot of buried fury. I know for me, I have always liked to imagine myself as being a calm, peaceful person, and for the most part, I am. However, I've also buried a lot in my life to try to keep the peace because I *wanted* to be a peaceful person. Recognizing and releasing that fury was an important step toward being able to hear my actual truth in so many parts of my life.

The Wisdom Within Chaos

There are many things that we cannot know within the structures that we are raised. They aren't taught in our schools, churches, or homes. These are the deep truths about spirituality, oneness, and the world. These are the truths for which spiritual seekers spend their entire lives seeking. We look to gurus, sacred texts, and spiritual communities for the answers. We know that there is something deep and important to find. Although we travel the world to meet amazing teachers and find community, we seldom find that magic that we seek so desperately… because, of course, it lies within us.

It lies in the mystery within. This is why it's difficult to find. It is in the chaos. It isn't in a neatly wrapped package. It doesn't follow the rules that we have been taught. It likely cannot even be expressed in words and doesn't follow the pathway of the logical mind.

It is in this mystery that our wild one lives. In fact, it is within this mystery that most of reality exists. It is quite a journey to embrace this idea — that it is actually impossible to understand the vast majority of reality. It is like the Taoist saying "The Tao that can be named is not the true Tao". This incredible mystery also lives within each one of us.

So, we must seek and explore the uncivilized parts of ourselves. We know that there is wisdom there. We trust it. This is one of the great ways in which we can learn to trust our emotional responses. This is where we watch what's happening with curious eyes, observing the world, but even more closely observing our soul's reaction to it.

There is wisdom there. There is magic in the mystery inside of each of us. It's who we truly are.

Our Supporting Masculine

So, how does our masculine serve the feminine in this instance? We are here to create. We are here to explore mystery. We are here to experience something new and different. How can our masculine side support that feminine chaos, mystery, and unknown that wants to be explored and expanded within us?

Let's say you want to swim with sharks. Well, this desire could get you killed. So, it may not be the best idea. But what if you were in a cage? What if you had excellent scuba gear and a boat? You could be put down among the sharks, in the cage, perfectly safe, still being able to commune with the sharks. This is a beautiful balance of wild desire and the safety and structure needed to have the experience.

MASCULINE STILLNESS

Another big way that the masculine balances our chaos is through stillness. We live in a chaotic world. There is always something unexpected going on somewhere. If it is not going on globally or nationally, our entire human body is chaotic. Our relationships are chaotic in that they are complex and filled with unknown mysteries.

I remember reading *The Book of Joy*, a conversation between the Dalai Lama and Desmond Tutu. Desmond Tutu said, "If human beings only understood how fragile they really were." Imagine if we realized that we are just one phone call away from our entire lives changing. This is the world we actually live in. We pretend that is not true which causes us a lot of suffering. We end up

STRUCTURE & CHAOS

working hard to fortify walls against what could happen, and then when something does happen, we are devastated.

Instead, we must develop our masculine stillness within to balance the external chaos. Within that stillness is great strength. Everything becomes calm. All the winds die down because now we are in the eye of the hurricane. We can hear guidance and our own thoughts. We can find ourselves within it. From here, we can hear what our next step is.

This is how we navigate a chaotic world.

It isn't that we have to solve everything on our own. Sometimes we sit and pray. Maybe a person's face pops into our mind, and we know we have to call them. It could be a friend that has important advice for us. It could be a practitioner who can help us. It could be anyone.

To do this, we have to be able to sit still. We have to access our masculine stillness in order to hear within the chaos.

Stillness Inside Emotions

This is especially important when we are unhappy. If we are hurting, and we know that we can access this strength of stillness, we are able to dive deeper into our emotions. The stronger our masculine is, the deeper we can dive into our anger, the more we can dive into our sadness, and the more we can admit to ourselves what the truth is within our chaos.

If we don't have that inner stillness, we will not be able to plumb the depths of our emotions without losing our balance. So, what is the answer? We practise specific pranayamas (breathing techniques) that help us rewire our minds and nervous systems. We meditate and do other things that help us feel peaceful. For some, it might be movements like wild dancing or running. If you are angry and a very physical person, you may just want to run and run and run. When you stop, the fury will have subsided, and you feel centred. For some people, it might be riding horses. For another, it could be playing music, walking in the woods, going for a swim, or walking their dog.

Whatever your stillness practice is, each time you do it will create a visceral pattern in your psyche that you will be able to default to the next time emotions and chaos threaten to overwhelm you. All you'll have to do is breathe deeply and find your centre within it.

Coming Back to Centre

When we have this beautiful, strong masculine within, we're not afraid of getting thrown off kilter. It is easier to stretch past our comfort zone in order to grow and experience something new because we know we have this strong lifeline within. We've experienced pulling ourselves out of difficult times before. Even if something does go wild and unexpected, we think, "It's okay. I may not like it, but I'll dive into it for a while to see what's in there. I know I'll come out of it. I have this strong centre. Everything will be okay."

Self-Care

In a world where there are a million moving parts, it makes sense that self-care is often silence, stillness, long baths, and walks in nature. The best self-care we have is beautiful structure, stillness, and quiet. It brings our life into balance. It's different, feels manageable, and gives us a space to hear guidance.

Imagine you are in a boat on the sea, and the waves are really big. You cannot stop the waves and the sea. What you do need to do is be able to go within and somehow get your bearings. Then you point your boat pointed in the direction you want to go, and trust that this is the right choice. That's all we do.

The world and the people in it can often feel like that sea. So many perspectives, power struggles, pain, desires, and confusion. This isn't going to change. However, if we can cultivate our inner stillness to find balance, it all becomes very doable and not so scary. We just have to find our bearing so that we know what the next step is.

This is the greatest self-love and self-care we can do: to cultivate the quiet within.

Structure & Chaos Together: The Meditation Journey

We often think that meditation is just about sitting quietly. In one way, it is very masculine because of its structure and stillness. It is also very feminine because we are just "being." Then, there is a dynamic dance between structure and chaos within meditation where we can discover amazing things about ourselves and about the world.

The point of meditation is not just masculine stillness. It is always a dance. Let's imagine that we are in a difficult time. We are feeling lost and want to come back into balance. We need to come back to our wholeness. So, we sit in a strong, masculine posture. This masculine stillness is important to balance the wildness and chaos that we feel inside. The more we are grieving, and the sadder we are, the stronger we need our structure to be. The act of creating this strong structure starts to affect us because when we feel out of control, we sometimes lose hope that we will ever feel better. The simple act of sitting in this posture sends a message to our body and mind: *We've got this.*

We then start to breathe deeply. This, first of all, shifts our nervous system out of fight-or-flight and into a more relaxed mode. We then start to drop our guards so that our feminine side can be felt. This is important because we often hold our breath in order to not feel what is going on. By breathing deeply, we begin the process of letting those feelings flow. By creating a masculine container within which they can be expressed, we can start to feel the sadness, the difficulty, the chaos, and the frustration. We can allow our truths to rise, for us to witness our emotions, and for healing to happen.

The key is to allow the dance. As the feelings rise, breathe deeply and let them flow while you press your sit-bones into the ground to strengthen your posture. As you strengthen the posture, your breath will become deeper and more emotions will be allowed to surface. Our masculine then hears and honours these inner truths, and the healing and integration process begins.

Your Personal Journey:

STRENGTHENING THE FEMININE

1. Do you enjoy the mystery within yourself? How do you access it? Ecstatic dance? Journaling? Doing wild things? Screaming? Deep meditation?
2. Do you fear the chaos inside and try to repress it? Or do you trust that there is wisdom there? How much chaos are you comfortable with?
3. Can you hear guidance and wisdom within your meditation practice? What have you heard before? What answers do you seek right now?
4. Is there a crazy idea inside of you that you would love to make happen? Has it been gnawing at you for a long time?
5. Do you love to be spontaneous? Are you good at creating a plan so that you can go wild?

STRENGTHENING THE MASCULINE

1. Do you have a daily meditation practice where you explore creating this masculine container for exploring within?
2. How do you come to stillness? Meditation, physical activity, artistic endeavours, time in nature? What kind of self-care can you do to support the wildness within you?
3. Did you have healthy structure growing up? Controlling parents? No structure? Where in your life have you experienced healthy structure that supported growth and new ideas? If you haven't, where could you create this now?
4. Are you comfortable holding space for others when they're hurting?
5. Do you enjoy the challenge of creating healthy structures and systems at work and in your personal life?

Chapter 7

Protector & Vulnerable

My book, "What if You Could Skip the Cancer?", is about my journey of learning to listen within and hear God or divine guidance. In the end, the lumps came out of the side of my breast, and I had a miraculous healing. One of the stories that didn't make it into the book was what happened the night before the lumps left.

I felt called to visit my friend, who is a very intuitive healer. I was in a dark and confused place and didn't know which end was up. I didn't know what to believe anymore. I didn't know what to take forward in my life or how to heal. It was a very confusing time.

She had some friends over when I got to her house. At one point, one of her friends (who also was into energy work and saw the world differently than most people) walked over to me and started gazing into my eyes. I just sat there because, if she saw something, I wanted to know. I was feeling so lost. She peered into my soul for a while and then said, "You sent your inner child away a long time ago because it wasn't safe."

You know those moments when everything lines up? I had never really thought about my inner child before that. I was a pretty strong person. I did my own thing. I took care of everybody. I never thought much about it. But at that moment, I knew she was right.

She looked at me and asked, "Do you want to bring her back?" I said, "Yes." She said, "Okay, I want you to envision a place that you are going to bring her back to, a place that she wants to come to." I closed my eyes and instantly, a vision appeared of an old library with wooden bookshelves

MASCULINE & FEMININE DYNAMICS

and a big wingback chair. My brain got in there and said, "That is stupid. What child would want to sit in a big wingback chair in a library?" But as much as my brain tried to create other scenarios that you would think a little girl would want to hang out in, they didn't work. I had to go back to the wingback chair in the dusty library.

As I opened my eyes, she asked, "Do you have the vision?" I said, "Yes." She said, "Now you have to make a promise to yourself that you'll keep her safe. She's allowed to go outside. She's allowed to play. But you always have to have her back, and you will always protect her.

Hmmm. This was a much bigger question. Because of my desire to be strong and independent, I had thrown my inner child to the wolves many, many times. I often put myself in positions where I was hurt. I didn't matter. It only mattered that other people's needs were met. My needs weren't important. It didn't matter if I was hurt. This was a big question. Was I willing to protect her?

In the end, I said yes. She said some magic words, and poof, there I was — little seven-year-old me sitting in the wingback chair.

Certainly, since then, there have been times when I've been a better protector of my inner child, and there have also been times that I still find myself throwing her to the wolves. But it definitely happens less and less.

This dynamic of the protector and the vulnerable exists within, as in this story, and with other people. When these dynamics are in separation, we fear feeling vulnerable and therefore our masculine rises too far and keeps everyone out and makes us never want to take chances. Or we ignore our true vulnerability (ignoring our feminine) and don't protect ourselves at all (having no masculine), forever "throwing ourselves to the wolves."

When our protector is connected to our vulnerability, the magnetic opposition of this polarity makes us strong. The more we feel the depth of our vulnerable truth, the bigger our protector becomes.

The bigger our protector is, the deeper we are able to dive into our vulnerability. We become stronger in both directions—more courageous and more insightful and wise.

How we experience this dynamic within ourselves definitely plays out in our relationships. So, let's explore what this looks like in our relationships with others.

Being the Protector

Protection is needed because there are many times when there are vulnerable ones around us needing protection. Vulnerability is part of being human, animal, or anything that can be in a vulnerable state and can't protect itself.

The domination paradigm we've lived within has created a lot of pain for innocent people. It has created a world of "haves" and "have-nots," and often, the "have-nots" need help. This paradigm also creates the "us" vs "them" dynamic. So, you end up with homophobia, racism, ageism, classism, sexism, and ableism. Because of these mentalities, inevitably, someone ends up being hurt. So, protection has become an important dynamic in our world.

This dynamic could be a parent defending their child. It could be a grown child defending a parent who is elderly and needs care. It could be a friend protecting another friend in the schoolyard. It could be someone rising up to protect a struggling minority. It could be a nurse advocating for a patient to make sure that they have the proper care.

Many feel an intense desire to protect the Earth. People have slept in trees for months to prevent deforestation. Many want to protect animals, whales, and the rainforest. The need is real, and the desire to protect is real. When everything is authentic and needed, and we rise into the protector role, a beautiful connection is made.

Parents Protecting Children

Children are vulnerable for most of their early lives. There is something very comforting for a child to know that their parents will always have their back and protect them no matter what. If a child doesn't have this growing up, they will often create protective barriers to the world that take decades (if ever) to come down.

Of course, protection doesn't mean not letting your children experience life. We must be careful not to project our fears onto our children and create such high walls of protection that our children can't experience anything. Our protectiveness is at its highest when they are the smallest. Each year, they must develop their own protection as their understanding of the world grows. The goal is for them to be complete, happy, and functional people. So, bit by bit, they will take up the awareness, develop their own protector-vulnerable balance, and protect themselves as needed.

Being Vulnerable

"The courage to be vulnerable is not about winning or losing. It's about the courage to show up when you can't predict or control the outcome."
BRENÉ BROWN

Vulnerability is not a weakness. Female animals in the wild require the protection of a mate only when they are caring for their young or birthing. This is not a weakness. It simply means that they are in no place to fight anyone off.

It is the same with us. Vulnerability is allowing an aspect of our psyche to need help and nurturance. This is not a constant state. It is a period in our life. It could be an hour, a week, or a year if we are going through difficult grief or a time of deep healing.

Yet vulnerability has been seen as a weakness, and perhaps for good reason. In the world of separation and domination, we are often preyed upon if we show weakness. Advertisers prey upon our fear of loneliness and desire for love. Churches prey upon our fear of what happens after we die. In some families, if you show your vulnerable side, parents and siblings would use that against you either at the time or later.

So, in many ways, being vulnerable has been a dangerous thing in the past. This danger has kept us quite separate from each other. So, it is a very important topic to look at.

Who Can We Be Vulnerable With?

> *"Do not give what is holy to the dogs;*
> *nor cast your pearls before swine,*
> *lest they trample them under their feet."*
> MATTHEW 7:6, New King James Bible

So, who can we be vulnerable with? We must always be sure that there is kindness and connection.

In all of these dynamics, we must actually be connected to each other. If you find a friend with whom you have a wonderful connection, the likelihood is that you will also feel safe to be vulnerable and honest with them. It is a relief to share who we truly are without worry.

We definitely want this in our romantic connections. These relationships are by definition "intimate." It isn't just that we are sexually active with this person. Intimacy is a deeper closeness than we might have with the average person or friend. It is the ability to truly share who we are, how we are feeling, and our truth at any moment without any kind of fear of judgment.

However, this too might be a challenge because many of us don't get into relationships with this in mind. Often, our life's training didn't require us to be emotionally solid or to live with full integrity. Plus, we weren't trained at all in healthy conflict resolution. Because most of us lack these skills, when things go awry in romantic relationships, unkind things can be said that push the other person away, and we no longer feel safe to be vulnerable.

When I wrote my book *Tantric Intimacy*, I didn't know how to start it because many couples I had worked with struggled to experience the deep intimacy they were seeking. This emotional safety that we're talking about was the greatest obstacle. Many had the belief that because they were married, they could act any way they wanted because their partner loved them and would never leave.

One of the first questions I would ask them is, "Can you be 100% kind to your partner for one week?" Over half of the answers were, "No." Some explained that sometimes they are tired and grumpy. Sometimes their partner pisses them off. Some even explained that they felt that that would be a boring relationship—to have to be nice to each other all of the time.

This is why we have a hard time being vulnerable. Many of us can't even imagine having a relationship that is safe enough to truly share in that way.

The first step is to develop *agape* for our partner. *Agape* is an Ancient Greek word meaning "God's love". Agape allows us to look at another person with full respect and awareness that they too are on a journey with many challenges and obstacles. As we also develop *agape* for ourselves, we become kinder within which translates into being kinder to everyone else.[2]

Challenges

Oftentimes, we are not living in situations where protection is needed, but we may have lots of leftovers as to how this dynamic has gone wrong in the past and how the dysfunction lives on in various ways.

OVERLY PROTECTIVE MASCULINE

We can see this in parents who protect their children to the point that the children have no freedom at all to explore the world. Every moment of the day is planned and accounted for. The children can't

---

[2] I discuss this at length in my book *Tantric Intimacy: Discover the Magic of True Connection*

walk anywhere alone. They can't hang out with their friends. They are coddled to the point of never developing any strength of their own. Obviously, sometimes we live in dangerous neighbourhoods where a child walking alone is truly unsafe. In this case, the protection is healthy.

Sometimes we are over-protective due to an ego desire to control, or it is done out of fear. The parent projects all their fears of the world onto their children and then tries to protect the children from those fears — whether the child has those fears or not.

This over-protectiveness can be seen in adult relationships as well. The person who prefers the masculine becomes controlling, wanting to know where their partner is at all times. They tell them that they can't do certain things or that they don't like certain friends of theirs. The masculine partner may check in with them throughout the day, making sure they always know what their partner is doing.

This is also where abuse is possible. The masculine partner becomes so controlling that the feminine partner is not allowed to think for themselves. The feminine partner stops going out with friends because their partner would rather have them at home. The feminine partner may not work because their partner wants to be the one to take care of them.

None of this is healthy because we are all meant to be independent, whole beings. No one should be in charge of anyone else. Everyone must have freedom of choice at all times.

False Feminine Vulnerability

In many parts of the world, women have historically been considered the "weaker sex", and because of this, they need someone to protect them. Obviously, this is ridiculous considering all that a woman is capable of. However, depending on our upbringing, we might realize that appearing vulnerable gets us a lot of attention. Feigning vulnerability is often used as a powerful tool to keep our partner's attention on us whenever we want it.

A woman once told me of a time when she was seeing a man who had a very busy schedule. He would often cancel their plans at the last moment because something came up. One day, he cancelled and she got really upset about it. She was feeling low and was looking forward to seeing him. Later, he messaged her, "How are you doing?" She replied, "Not very well actually. I am not in a great place and was really looking forward to seeing you."

The next thing she knew, he was at her door. He had dropped everything to come to be with her. As he walked in the door, he could see that she was visibly upset. He said, "Oh, I'm so sorry. I want you to know that I am always here for you. There is nothing that would ever stop me from coming to see you!" She stared at him thinking, *"Ummm, there are always a million things that stop you from coming to see me. What are you talking about?"*

She had learned something about him. She would become a priority in his life as long as she was upset and needed him. She realized that if she was self-sufficient and didn't need him, he would just go about his business, and she would drop lower on his priority list.

What should she do? If she wanted to see him more often, she would have to maintain a relatively upset and vulnerable state. It wouldn't be true vulnerability. It would be an act, but she would get the connection with him that she truly desired. This, of course, is manipulation. It is avoiding the real issues in their relationship and her lack of inner balance and happy life outside of him. But you can see the temptation to just stay a little weak all of the time.

Wanting to Make Our Partner Feel Strong

Sometimes, the feminine partner will pretend to be weaker than they actually are in order to make the masculine partner feel strong. If the masculine partner has been emasculated in their lives or doesn't feel good about themselves, they may not feel like they can take the masculine role. This could result in the relationship having no spark and no polarity. So, the feminine will play small hoping that the masculine will feel big. Unconsciously we hope that they will feel so masculine, the masculine-feminine dynamics of our relationship will become alive and exciting.

Of course, it doesn't work. It doesn't change the fact that they have been emasculated. This must be looked at. Their true strength is all they have. They have inner work to do outside of the relationship. And for the feminine partner, playing small can lead to depression and existential boredom. The act can only last for so long before they will have to return to their actual size.

We Are Not Always the Protector or Vulnerable

"Being vulnerable is the only way to allow your heart to feel true pleasure."
BOB MARLEY

This is one of the dynamics where it is easy to get stuck in the masculine or feminine role. We might identify masculine as someone who is big, strong, and a protector. However, unless we are actually protecting someone, we are not masculine. We are just ourselves, ideally balanced — both masculine and feminine.

Similarly, being meek, quiet, and subservient has historically been defined as being feminine. This is not a healthy state to live in. We are all meant to be whole. Unless we are being attacked, overpowered, or we are unable to stay safe because we have children or others in our care, we are not weak, nor do we need protection from anyone.

The challenge is that if I like being the protector, I may never allow myself to be vulnerable. On the flipside, I may be attached to always being in the vulnerable role, never accessing my own strength. In both cases, there's no inner balance or true strength.

When we are attached to one polarity, we will surround ourselves with friends and intimate partners who are also stuck, only in the opposite polarity. If you are attached to being in the vulnerable role, you may only attract people who are "ever-protectors". They will feel it's their job to tell you what you can and can't do. They will say that they are just keeping you safe and taking care of you, and the vulnerable partner will be happy because they will love the attention. However, depending on their partner, they may lose all autonomy. They will default to what their partner says, and because they always want to be in that vulnerable role, they will keep making decisions that are not from a place of strength.

It is the same for people who always want to be in the protector role. They will only find people who are needy and always wanting a protector. They don't find equals. They always want to be the white knight coming in to save the damsel in distress (all genders). It feels okay for the same reason — they want the connection. Even though neither person is coming into their wholeness, the ever-protector has someone to protect and care for, and the ever-vulnerable one has someone who cares for them.

There are many reasons why we may want to identify with either the protector or the protected one. Maybe the ever-masculine person had to protect their younger siblings from a parent as a child. Maybe they have past lives where they were soldiers, and this is just a pattern they are repeating. Or perhaps it is scary to be vulnerable and look at the pain inside, so it is easier to just stay in the masculine so you never have to look at it.

If you are attached to being the vulnerable one, maybe this was the only way you got attention as a child. Maybe the strong ones were left to fend for themselves. However, if you were hurting, sick, or confused, your parents would naturally spend more time with you. Maybe being vulnerable in the schoolyard attracted kids to protect you, and it made you feel special. Or maybe it is just something picked up from Hollywood and romance novels that to be the damsel in distress is very romantic and emotionally rich.

When this dynamic plays out this way, it is total co-dependence. We need to have this other person, or else we don't feel whole. This creates many issues in the relationship, and as much as we may desire the connection, it will not be healthy. The ever-protector will keep flexing their control muscles and never admit their vulnerability, therefore, acting unconsciously in the relationship. The ever-vulnerable will quietly rebel against the control doing things "against their partner's wishes" because their soul doesn't want to be controlled.

You can just imagine the constant drama that would ensue and build upon itself.

The Question of Chivalry

"I'm an old soul that believes in chivalry, romance and love."
ADRIAN MICHAEL

Chivalry has gotten a bad rap ever since the women's equality movement. After years of being treated as a non-person and a long fight to be treated equally, the last thing many women want is to have a man open a door for them. It's seen as a message that they are still weaker than men, and they don't like it.

Including chivalry in this book could be a little risky. And yet, when our masculine partner does that little extra to open our doors, carry our bags, and be a little bit more attentive than others, something in our heart opens and feels loved. Magnetism increases. So, it's an important topic to look at.

Originally, chivalry was a social code of knightly conduct. It included duties to countrymen, duties to God, and duties to women. Let's look at that last one.

It was the idea that the knight must serve his lady. He was asked to be especially gentle and gracious with her. It's natural to wonder why this was a rule of the knights. However, if we think about what life was like back in the 1200s when the code of chivalry was developed, men weren't so kind to women as a general rule. Women were often treated like slaves, brood-mares, and much worse by their families and husbands. A knight was considered to be better than the average man, and therefore, more was expected of him—especially in his treatment of women.

MASCULINE & FEMININE DYNAMICS

When we consider the spirit of this, it becomes very beautiful for a masculine partner to open a door for the feminine partner, carry their bags, and stand in the way of danger. The masculine doesn't do this because the feminine is weak. He wants to protect her because he loves her. It is much more like wanting to do something for their queen than doing it because the feminine can't do something or is weak in any way.

I've had people argue that this isn't right because it is so one-sided. Yes, this is true, and it is intentional. We are studying the magnetism of the dance between masculine and feminine energies. It is about what empowers each person, increases the magnetism, which then leads to the union. When the masculine partner stands up, and chivalrously lays down their metaphorical coat across a puddle for their partner to walk on, both partners' desired magnetism is increased. Could the feminine partner hold the umbrella or open the door? Sure. But it has a different energy about it. The masculine partner could appreciate it, feel emasculated, or feel nothing at all. It's not wrong by any means. It just won't increase the energy of our polarity in the ways that we are seeking.

There are arguments like, "Oh, no. Women are equal to men. They are equally strong and equally powerful." Of course, this is true. Equality never should have been a question. However, when the masculine partner gets to protect and care for their feminine partner, confidence rises inside of them, and the feminine feels loved and cared for. It is never about the feminine being weak or needy. The feminine could absolutely do it herself. That's why it's special.

In much of the world, we are living in a time of gender equality. No one has to hold an umbrella over us, carry the bags, or open the door for anyone. Nobody has to do anything. Everyone has choice. When we choose to do it, it creates connection. If we choose to not accept anyone's help, we stay separate. But when we choose to polarize and to play with chivalry, we can create a truly beautiful bond.

Protector & Vulnerable Within

How do we bring this protector and vulnerable dynamic into balance within ourselves? How can we be our own protectors? How can we feel free to access our deepest vulnerability and connect with who we truly are?

THE SPIRIT OF OUR INNER PROTECTOR

One day, I was co-teaching a class with my daughter about self-love and boundaries. She was twenty-five years old at the time. I was telling the room how I had always struggled with my self-worth and had a hard time setting strong boundaries with others.

My daughter looked at me and said, "It's interesting that you struggle with that. With us [her and her brother], you were always such a mama bear. We knew that you would always protect us no matter what. We knew that you would always create healthy boundaries around us so that no one could hurt us. Maybe you just need to love yourself as much as you loved us."

Mic drop.

This is what is behind our inner protector—self-love. It is the sentinel at the door who loves us. He keeps anyone and anything at bay who might harm us in any way.

Why? Because he loves us so much.

SAYING NO

It is our protector who says *no* to others when needed. When someone says, "Can you do this for me?" We close our eyes and ask what our inner child says. If the answer is *no*, then a clear, "No, thanks," is given.

This is a huge deal because many of us have been raised that we mustn't disappoint anyone. Therefore, we may say yes just to keep others happy. But who suffers for that? We do.

However, our protector won't allow us to suffer so that someone else doesn't feel bad. He loves us too much. Knowing that our deepest, most vulnerable self will always be protected brings incredible peace inside. We always know we will have our own back. It is a beautiful feeling.

Not only do we have this quiet inner peace, but we also have more courage to step into scary situations. We are usually afraid that we won't protect ourselves—that we will say "yes" when we want to say "no"—that we won't walk away when we should. However, if we always know that our protector is strong and devoted to our feminine, we will have the courage to do things that we never thought we could because we always have our own back.

Healthy Boundaries

Many people struggle with not having strong boundaries. They are open and vulnerable. This can be a good thing because it makes us available and able to connect with others. However, when our masculine is not strong, then we fall out of balance, and we tend to get trampled. It is like people perpetually coming into your home and making a mess and breaking things. You need someone at the door who explains the rules of the house and kicks them out if they break the rules... and then doesn't allow them back in again.

But this protector is not a brute. The protector intimately understands the desires of the vulnerable heart that he is protecting. It is not a jail. This is where you must have full communication between the masculine and feminine. The heart has experiences. The protector considers these and then takes action.

You can imagine how this can go awry.

What if your heart is broken too many times? Your masculine rises up to protect you so that you won't be hurt again—so you don't let anyone in. When the pain is raw, this is a good thing. We must create space in order to heal. Then the heart must talk to the protector about opening up again when it is time. Hearts don't want to be alone forever. The masculine must honour each new state of being as we heal.

Similarly, the heart must also listen to the protector sometimes. Let's say that you have ended an abusive relationship. After a time, your heart might want to forget about the past and get back together. However, the protector remembers and wants to keep you safe. This is where it is a good idea for the feminine to listen to the masculine. The protector can't help you if you keep letting yourself get hurt over and over again. Eventually, the protector will just give up, and unbalanced chaos will ensue.

Embracing Our Vulnerability Within

When we have a strong inner protector, we easily allow ourselves to feel everything within us. We can feel the happy moments, sad ones, strong times and weak ones.

However, sometimes we pretend that things don't bother us and are always "fine" even when we are not, limiting our experience of everything because we are blocking important messages about our lives.

Maybe there were experiences from our childhood that were very difficult, and we locked them away so that we didn't feel that pain any longer. Although they were removed from our conscious awareness, they still affect us. They may stop us from connecting deeply with others. They might stop us from manifesting our desires for fear of exposure to criticism. They may cause a lack of self-love which affects us all day long. At some point in our adult life, we have to unpack those experiences and let them into our conscious mind, and the only way to do that is to feel those vulnerable emotions.

Vulnerability comes up in our current experiences as well. We may be chatting with our parents, and they say something hurtful. If we don't allow ourselves to actually feel the sting of their words, our inner masculine will not be called upon to protect us and respond properly. Instead, we will bury our vulnerable truth and continue to allow them to treat us this way.

MASCULINE & FEMININE DYNAMICS

Vulnerability is allowing ourselves to see the reality of any situation. We may have a job that pays well and is well-respected by others, but deep down, it is silently killing us. We don't actually want to go to work any longer, and we are beginning to resent our children, partner, and everyone whom this job supports. If we don't listen to and value this vulnerable truth, we may never make the changes needed to start feeling better about our lives and everyone we love.

Vulnerability also gives you space when you need it. In my previously mentioned healing journey, I was sick with lumps growing in my breasts. This was only four years after my mom had died of breast cancer. The whole story can be found in my book *What if You Could Skip the Cancer?*, but what's important here is that once I realized I wasn't going to go the medical route, and I was following an inner path, I cut myself off from almost everyone in my life. My journey was to start listening to my own truths and honour my deep and vulnerable self. If I shared too much with my friends and family, they would all have an opinion. They would have fears. They would want to "help," and I definitely didn't have the energy to field their questions and try to make them feel okay about the choices I was making.

My masculine stood in the gap for me and created a great space between me and most other people. He gave me permission to not share everything. I was too fragile. I was trying to hear deep truths that I had buried my whole life. I could barely explain them to myself, and I knew that my inner focus and resolve could crumble if I was pressed too hard from the outside.

Within that masculine protection, I was able to dive deeply into myself. I was able to go into corners that perhaps no women in my family had ever been able to go (they had all died of cancer like my mom). I was allowed to go into the scary places.

I was able to go there because I knew that I was totally safe and protected.

Your Personal Journey:

STRENGTHENING THE FEMININE

1. Are you able to be vulnerable with yourself? Does vulnerability feel safe for you? Are there experiences in your past where this wasn't safe?
2. Do you trust your inner masculine to protect you? Do you listen to him?
3. Are you comfortable being vulnerable with others? Is it okay to show your soft side? Are there particular people with whom you like being vulnerable?
4. Do you enjoy it when someone is chivalrous toward you? Are you able to accept this from them?

STRENGTHENING THE MASCULINE

1. Do you stand in the gap for your vulnerable self when out in the world?
2. Are you over-protective of your inner child? Do you need to let others see her more often?
3. Do you easily say "no" if that is the truth? Do you easily hold strong boundaries?
4. Do you easily step into the protector of others when needed?
5. Do you enjoy being chivalrous? Are there any negative ideas about this that you'd love to clear up? Where did they come from?

Chapter 8

Leading & Following

In 2006, I opened a dance studio with a man who was an incredible dancer and teacher.

At the time, my husband didn't feel comfortable dancing. He's a great dancer now, but back then, when we went to weddings, I would just "back-lead" him, which means that it would look like he was leading, but I was actually the one moving us around. Since I always wanted to dance with him, I became really good at back-leading.

Now I had opened a dance studio with a man who had been dancing for over thirty years. There would be no back-leading here. I would have to learn to follow. Trying to back-lead him would be like trying to move a wall. If I tried, he would just look at me, smile, and say, "Katrina, just relax. Let me lead."

It didn't take long before I started to relax. Once I did, I was able to pick up his cues more easily. I relaxed my guard and connected more deeply with him. It became more and more enjoyable until the day came when the magic happened. I finally dropped all of my guards, and we fell into true union. My feet no longer touched the floor. My head tipped back, and everything went soft and wonderful. I would become so blissful when this happened that he would often laugh at me saying, "Come back, Katrina! Come back to Earth!"

This feeling of total surrender brings you to the most ecstatic floating space. It's not just enjoyable. It is so much more. It is the bliss of total and complete union.

The Joy of Leading

There are many examples of wonderful leading and following. However, the historical desire for power has shown us leaders and rulers who simply want control, which is not leading. This history has caused us to fear "leaders" and the idea of being one. As a natural consequence, we often struggle to follow as well.

Some people are born leaders. These people have vision. They have integrity, and we love to follow them. They have no need for power or control over anyone. Everyone acts within their own choice and truth.

Bosses can be great leaders when they genuinely know and care about their team. They know the strengths and weaknesses of their employees, and they organize what needs to be done so that everyone gets the assignment for which they are best suited. They enjoy the pressure and challenges of responsibility. It makes them stronger and helps them grow. Their people know this and love being a part of their team.

Kinds of Leaders

There are two kinds of leaders. The first is a thought leader. These are people like Martin Luther King Jr and Gandhi. They are fully connected to the Divine, they have great ideas, and they make things happen. As they walk forward in their vision, people want to follow. This leader has more of a teacher-student dynamic. They offer ideas, and the followers listen and absorb. They aren't directly connected to their followers. It is more the followers who are connected to them.

The second type of leader's role is to guide the others in a group of two or more. One person makes the plan and the others follow. This could be a team leader in a business, the coach of a sports team, your dance partner, or a guide through the Himalayas. Through this division of roles, a beautiful, cohesive unit is formed that brings everyone to a great experience.

Many people are born leaders, and they just rise to this position throughout their lives. You can see this in children on the playground when they are all hanging around wondering what to do. What game do they want to play? There might be a child who says, "Hey, I've got an idea. Let's do this. Okay, see that hill over there? That's the castle, and we have to get there through this forest…" and the kids all say, "Oh, yeah. Awesome!"

These are people whom others just want to follow. There is no loss of power. The other kids heard a great idea and said, "That'll be fun. I want to play!" After that, everyone contributes to the game. Who came up with the idea is irrelevant because everyone is now having fun playing.

Leadership is Not a Hierarchy

"A leader is best when people barely know he exists, when his work is done, his aim fulfilled, they will say: we did it ourselves."
LAO TZU

Historically, within the domination patriarchy, the leader is at the top of a hierarchy, but this is not a masculine role. It is just a power position in a world of separation. Instead, we see the leader as playing a role in a group. They are connected to everyone, and their role is to lead the whole to whatever experience they are seeking.

On a project team, the only goal of a good leader is to get the job done. The best way to do that is to have everyone in the room working within their skill set with the freedom to create according to their gifts. In fact, a natural leader can't help themselves from assessing every person as they are introduced. They will instantly know what the gifts are of every single person on the team. They will look around and think, "Okay. He is the people person. She is the one doing the math. This person knows the science. That one gets the tech." From there, they just put the puzzle pieces together. Everyone is seen and happy.

MASCULINE & FEMININE DYNAMICS

COACHES & COMMUNITY LEADERS

True leaders often show up as brilliant sports coaches. They are the ones who see the big picture. They look at all the players and instantly figure out the team. They notice the interactions between them. They know who the aggressive and the quiet ones are. They also know how to tailor the training so that everybody thrives because their goal is the success of the whole.

A dysfunctional coach wants the team to win no matter what. The kids are just pawns in their ego game. Well, the kids instinctively won't want to play for that person, and you'll see a lot of dysfunction in the team. There will be fighting and parents yelling all the time. It will be no fun for anyone.

However, for a good coach whose goals are building up the kids' character, skills, and ability to work and play as a team, those kids will listen because energy doesn't lie. The kids know that this person cares and the parents know too. If any parents get out of line, that coach just looks at them and asserts, "We are in this for the whole team. You can decide whether you want your child to be part of this or not. But we have no prima donnas, and we don't pick on the kids who are struggling. We are here for the whole. That is my job as the leader."

We often respond very positively to that because we feel safe. We know that our kids are being seen, and perhaps, although we are adults, we ourselves are learning how to play with others.

These leaders are often born that way. They have a natural gift of seeing the big picture, all the pieces, and how to put them together to get to the finish line. At the same time, if someone found themselves in a leadership position, and it wasn't necessarily their gifting, they could certainly learn. They just have to know that their job is not to have power over others. Their job is to bring everybody together, according to their gifts.

In the community, we always find these leaders too. They will have great visions for projects that happen in the community. You can always tell if it is only about them getting their name on it versus someone who is actually part of the community and wants to help out. Maybe that person helps with time, skills, or money. One way or the other, they just want to enjoy the connections that are possible.

Leading in Couple's Dancing

When we dance by ourselves on the dancefloor, it is about the union of our bodies and the music. If a group of people are on the dancefloor having fun, they will each be dancing in their own way with their own inspiration and moves—each one very individual and separate.

If we want to do ballroom or Latin dance, the goal is for two people to create a single unit dancing together. Therefore, we must split into our polarities. We must each become either feminine or masculine. If we stay separate, we will just be co-dancing. We might be touching and dancing similar steps, but there won't be true union. There will tend to be a push-pull happening as each person tries to get the other to dance their way.

Instead, one person is the leader (masculine), and the other is the follower (feminine). The first thing to be clear about is that no one is in control of the other person. Although the leader is choosing the next step, the follower has their own flair. The feminine also has full choice whether they want to continue dancing with this leader, and ironically, a good leader makes their choices based on their feminine follower.

I am going to use a male/female example, but it could be anyone. Imagine you are at a wedding, and one of your cousins is an incredible dancer. Later, at the dance, an amazing salsa song comes on. Your cousin looks across the dancefloor and sees a woman in a sexy dancing dress. Based on her dress and shoes (all dancers wear specific dancing shoes), he figures that she knows how to dance. So, he walks across the floor to ask her to salsa with him.

As they begin dancing, he starts out slowly, feeling her out. How much dance has she done? What style did she learn? Or is it just a beautiful dress and shoes? He leads her in a few steps and realizes that she is an exceptional dancer. She knows all kinds of moves and is an amazing follower. He continues to try new steps and plays with what's possible between them. She realizes that he is a great leader and she relaxes more into the following role. He notices that she has relaxed and is trusting him, so he tries some fancier moves. They dance and become like one in an incredible, whirling experience. They are truly a sight to behold!

All too soon, that song ends. He thanks her for the dance, and as he's about to sit down, a beautiful waltz comes on. He sees his grandma over in the corner and heads over to ask her to dance, and Grandma is happily led out onto the dancefloor. How does he dance with her? Does he dance in the same way he danced with the salsa dancer? No. He shortens his step. He does slower moves. He bases his lead on Grandma's dance experience, her physical ability, and whatever steps make her smile.

There is great joy here. The leader, because he loves to dance and experience the union of the dance, has just as much fun dancing with Grandma as dancing with the salsa dancer. It is the union that creates joy and happiness.

For him, the challenge to lead is exciting. Every partner he dances with that night will be different. Each one will have a different feel, ability, and will enjoy different things. His thrill is in applying what he knows to all of those unique situations.

How to Be a Great Leader

> *"In Ojibwe and Cree culture,*
> *'Leadership' didn't mean power;*
> *It meant caring."*
> TANYA TALAGA

There are a few main characteristics of a leader that can create an incredible union.

Connection

The leader must always be connected to the follower—this is at work, sexually, in the family, and all the time. It is always about connection. The leader knows the value of this. They know the pleasure, joy, and happiness that happen when humans connect.

I love fixing up houses. When I was a child, my mom and dad did all kinds of renovations, and they were good leaders. They were good at saying, "Okay, today, we are going to get this done. Katrina, you go do this…" and my sisters would get jobs as well. They would always give us jobs we liked. To this day, we all love painting and renovating our homes. Once you experience the joy of a group working together with a good leader, you know the value of it.

Whenever you're in the position of leader, the goal is always connection. None of this works without it. If we personally struggle with connection, that is where we have to start. Why do we struggle to be open? Why do we have guards up? These are things we have to work on. If we are unable to connect with others, we must get to the root of that resistance and practise slow and gentle connections in a safe context because this connection is the foundation that we must have.

Surrender to the Whole

As much as we are leading and choosing the next steps, our first step is surrendering to the combined experience. Being a leader isn't making the call regardless of who else is in the group or who our partner is. We read our partner or group and then listen within to know what to do.

Imagine that you are at work, and you're the leader of a team. There is a certain surrendering of the ego, a surrender of whatever ideas you once had. You know what the goal of the group is. Then you surrender to what's possible, however the dynamics flow. That is very different from imposing an idea on the group and making it happen from the top down.

This surrender of the leader is a huge deal, and perhaps, as in life, humility is always the answer. We must remember that "leader" is just a role we are playing. Today, I get to be the leader. Tomorrow, I might be the follower. So, today, as the leader, I will surrender to that role.

BEING TRUSTWORTHY

I used to teach wedding couples how to dance. Once, a couple came to me to learn their first dance. The bride was a spitfire and in charge of everything. The groom was a quiet guy who didn't really say much. This was one of the great challenges in teaching them to dance because he really didn't seem to care, and she really wanted him to.

One of the challenges in teaching couples is that they will dance in the same way they navigate their relationship. If there's a power struggle between them, they will have the same struggle on the dance floor. In the first few sessions, there is always a bit of a learning curve for the teacher as some aspects of the dynamic simply don't work. Eventually, the truth will come out that there is an issue in their relationship getting in the way of learning the dance. So, it is often a gentle process going forward.

With this couple, I was struggling to get him to lead. He just acted like, "Yeah, whatever she wants." And I would say, "No, you have to lead. She gets to follow here."

After a few classes, they were at the place where it was time for him to lead and her to follow. He was confident enough. He knew the moves, he could hear the beat, and he knew the choreography. It was time to make this happen.

Well, I had a stage set up in the corner of my studio for a concert that was happening that night. It was made of rough-cut lumber, and the edges were a little sharp. It was a bit of an obstacle for dancing, but a good leader would simply lead their partner around it. I told him ahead of time to watch out for it because the bride-to-be was going to close her eyes so she could focus completely on following.

I said to him, "You are 100% in control. You are responsible for her. She can't see where she's going." In ballroom dance, the woman is nearly always walking backward. The leader has to be in control and trustworthy to make sure that she's not going to bang into anything.

I started the music, and they began the choreography. He was being his nonchalant self. However, she was really struggling to relax into the following role.

As I watched them dance, I saw them getting closer and closer to that stage, which was only a few inches tall. She was in heels. If she backed into it, she would scratch the back of her ankles.

What did he do? He backed her right into the stage so that she hurt the back of her ankle and then he laughed. I stopped him and said, "Why did you do that? She was trusting you." He said, "Yeah, but it was funny, wasn't it?"

I said, "No. You hurt her."

"I know. I know. But it's funny. I mean, she had her eyes closed and everything."

This is why she couldn't trust him as a leader. Deep down, she already knew this because of their relationship. She didn't want to admit it, but as soon as she closed her eyes and had to be truly vulnerable, she knew she was in trouble because he just wasn't trustworthy.

This is very important. If we want someone to be able to join us and follow, they need to know that they can close their eyes and trust us. This is often more responsibility than we are used to or want. Sometimes we want to be like children. We don't want to be responsible. In the case of this groom, he wanted the status of "being the man," but had no interest in actually acting in any masculine way.

Enjoying Following

Because of the separation and domination that we have experienced, following is often hard to step into. Historically, it often meant a loss of personal power. We have seldom experienced the beautiful union that can happen between lead and follow where it is simply a meeting of equals taking on different roles so that we can unite and experience bliss.

This is a challenge for anyone who has ever been forced to do anything they didn't want to do. This could be from childhood, school, work or relationships. It can be in all genders and demographics—anyone who was ever oppressed by anyone else. We need to understand our past if we are struggling to follow now. We don't have to stay there. We just want to be aware of it so that we can integrate it, heal, and learn to follow because it is so joyful.

Let's talk about some aspects of following.

FOLLOWING MUST BE VOLUNTARY

Following must always be something you want to do. It is the magnetism of the masculine that makes you think, "Oh, I would like to follow this person." In a job, it's knowing, "Yes, I would love to work for that person. I love what they are doing. I know they are good to their employees. I would enjoy working there."

There is a voluntariness, a desire, and a want to follow. It is finding out that someone's a great dancer and saying, "I would love to dance with that person because I know they are a great lead." It is the desire to be with someone intimately. As soon as you know and feel that they are paying attention to you, you effortlessly want to surrender to the experience.

If someone has to say to you, "Trust me. It's okay," this is a big red flag. If you don't feel inside of you that this is a safe place, then we have to be honest about that. We live in a world where there has been a lot of forced submission and forced following. We have often been taught to ignore that wisdom inside that knows what's a good idea and what isn't. You should never have to be told to trust someone. Whether we trust someone or not is a primal self-protection instinct. Either you do, or you don't. Maybe they will be different in the future, and the trust will be automatic, but how we feel right now is all we know for sure.

Holding Your Frame

In dancing, it is important to "hold our frame" so that we don't collapse into the other person. Although we are going to dance together, and the goal is union, we each still stand in our own centre. We don't allow our bodies to collapse into each other. We connect with relatively tense arms so that we can feel each other's lead and follow, but we remain our own person.

You can imagine how important this is in relationships. Even if we desire a beautiful union, we are still our own people. If I collapse my frame, I disappear as a person, and following is not about disappearing. It is about bringing all of both of you together and making something greater.

This is a possibility that many in the older generations didn't get the chance to experience. We were taught for centuries that in marriage, we "cleave together to become one." However, it was usually the woman who simply joined the man's life. After getting married, I received mail addressed to "Mrs. Wayne Bos." This was supposed to be me. I had decided to change my last name to his. Perhaps, in some people's minds, I had also changed my first name to his. Or perhaps I didn't even have a first name. I was just his wife.

This is an old idea that, hopefully, is no longer around by the time you read this book. But it is interesting to consider this in all of the feminine roles we play in all genders.

Being Able to Both Lead and Follow in Life

> *"Great leaders are willing to follow.*
> *Leadership is a dance, not a parade."*
> JESSE LYN STONER

I used to own a train station called East Street Station in Goderich, Canada. I had renovated it into a community centre where I did all of my teaching and often had guest teachers come in to teach on other interesting topics.

There was one man who used to come to teach all kinds of business topics. He was a natural-born leader with a huge personality and a big, booming voice. He was incredibly strong in that leadership role with a truly commanding presence.

I had created a class about the connection between spirituality and health, and was so surprised to see that this man had signed up for it as a student. I wondered how this was going to go. Was he going to passive-aggressively take over the class? Sometimes when people are attached to being in a leadership role, they are perpetually putting up their hand just to draw attention to themselves. Often, they are not really asking questions. They are simply taking the floor, which can be really distracting when you are teaching.

On the first day, he walked into the class, sat down in the second row and completely blended in with everyone else. This larger-than-life human I normally witnessed had disappeared. He became a student. Fully listening. Fully receiving. It was the most amazing lesson for me, to watch him morph into a follower instead of a leader, just for the day. The next day, he'd become the leader he needed to be.

This is an ability that is important in all of the dynamics. The better we are at receiving, the better we are at giving. The more vulnerable we can be, the better protector we are, and so on. In this man's case, his ability to fully polarize into the feminine allowed him to fully polarize into an even better and more effective leader.

Fully Understanding the Other Polarity

Sometimes, while teaching a couple to dance, I would get them to switch roles. This is for dancers who want to perfect their lead or follow. Let's say that Dancer A normally loves to lead, and Dancer B is normally the follower.

First, Dancer A has to learn the follower's steps, which are often the opposite of what they are doing and Dancer B must learn the leader's steps.

Then Dancer A must relax and trust Dancer B to lead them. They must receive the cues for the next step without anticipating them or planning what they would like to do next in their head. They soon learn that there are many muscles inside of them that must release in order to be able to trust Dancer B's lead. They somehow have to fully relax and enjoy following.

They also learn how confusing the leader's cues might be. When ballroom dancing, the follower might only get a cue like the leader raising their arm which might indicate a spin. Their foot might lead them a bit to the side indicating a side-step. If these cues aren't clear, the follower is left guessing, and they are no longer in union. New leaders are often frustrated when their partner isn't picking up on their cues. But once they have a chance to try to follow someone else's lead, they realize that they need to be much clearer the next time they are the leader.

Similarly, when Dancer B has to lead, they discover how challenging that can be. They realize that they are suddenly responsible for two people. They not only have to figure out their own feet, but they must also guide and lead their partner. They discover that they also must strengthen some muscles inside to allow them to be strong and confident. They have to really focus while they are learning to get the leading steps and partner cues perfect so that they can become second nature. Once they are second nature, then they can relax into the dance, the lead, and the bliss of the union. But initially, the dancers need serious focus.

This is so powerful to do in life. If you tend to be a follower, taking an opportunity to practise being a good leader gives you such a different perspective than always being the one able to criticize those making the decisions. Similarly, if you are always in control and driving the bus, taking a course with a teacher you respect and just relaxing into the role of student is not only relaxing and nourishing, but you will become a much better leader yourself.

Your Personal Journey:

Strengthening the Feminine

1. Do you enjoy following a good leader?
2. Have you found many people who were good leaders in your life whom you could happily follow? Who were some great leaders? Who was not?
3. Are there experiences in your life that have created blocks in you that stop you from recognizing a good leader and relaxing into the following?
4. Are you good at "holding your frame" in life, or do you tend to collapse into others?

Strengthening the Masculine

1. Who have been great leaders in your life? What made them great? How did it feel to follow their lead?
2. Who weren't good leaders? Are there people in your life who just like to control but are pretending to lead?
3. Do you like to lead? Is this a comfortable role for you? Are you good at it? Or does it end up being more about control? (If it is, then this becomes an interesting journey of discovery to find out why.)
4. Can you easily morph from leader to follower depending on the situation

SECTION III

Finding Balance Within

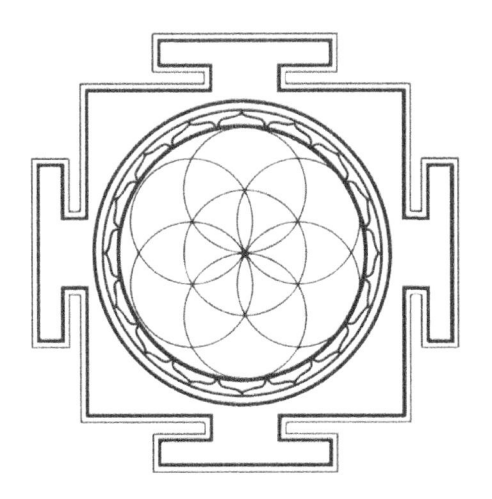

Chapter 9

Inner Happiness

*"The union of feminine and masculine energies
within the individual
is the basis of all creation."*
SHAKTI GAWAIN

It is our inner masculine-feminine balance that makes us feel alive. We feel potent. We feel like we matter and that we are supposed to be here. We manifest what we desire. We feel strong because our inner protector loves our vulnerable selves. We receive what we desire because we give to ourselves. The more we rest, the more we can create. The more we create, the deeper we rest. The more logic and structure we have, the more we can be free and spontaneous.

When we are disconnected inside, we often become stagnant— similar to what happens in a disconnected relationship. But when we have this dynamic balance within us, we can't help but bring it to all the relationships in our life. Every relationship we have will soon follow the same pattern that we have within.

This is good news because it means that we can always do something to find happiness. It isn't about other people changing. It is about us shifting inside and finding that aliveness ourselves. Then, we can just invite other people to the party.

Meeting Our Two Sides

In my early forties, I was recently divorced, single, and quite lonely. I had moved to Toronto and, with a population somewhere around six million, dating was a lot easier than in the small town in which I had been living. Needless to say, I started dating a lot.

After a few months of this new freedom, my seventeen-year-old daughter looked at me and said, "Mom, it's weird. It's like you have this shadow of a man beside you, and you are just looking for someone to fill it." I had been married for twenty years. I was so accustomed to having a partner, I didn't know how to be whole unto myself. And even before I was married, all I cared about was finding "that special someone." So yes, I was desperately seeking someone to fill that void.

I also realized that men were my favourite drug that made me feel better when I was sad and feeling lost. Between these realizations and the fact that I was working on healing long-standing anemia, I decided to go celibate. I realized that how I related to men (whether I was married to them or not) drained my energy. To get better, I needed to plug all such leaks. Whether I liked it or not, celibacy was the answer. I didn't like it. But alas, this was to be my new adventure.

So how could I be whole unto myself? How could I get to a place where I didn't need a man to make me feel whole? How could I draw that shadow back into my being and feel complete again?

The answer was a vision of having two sides—masculine and feminine. I was the feminine, and whoever I was seeking was the masculine. To be whole, I needed to have that masculine within me instead of seeking it outside.

I asked myself, "What would my favourite partner be like? What is it that he would add to my life? What is it that I'd want him to do?"

So, I decided to become my own best boyfriend.

INNER HAPPINESS

I looked at the dynamics of masculine and feminine, the giving, the receiving, the structure, the chaos, the protection, the vulnerability, and I started asking myself certain questions. "Does my inner masculine give to my inner feminine? If my inner feminine needs something or desires something, do I give that to her?"

I realized that I didn't, and I had to start. I had to start giving her what she desired and start making her happy.

Sometimes it was as simple as wanting to go out for dinner. My feminine might say, "Oh, I'd love to try out that new Italian restaurant." It was interesting how often I fought with myself. My masculine side might say, "We don't need that. It's too expensive." Or he would say, "Sure, that is a great idea!" and then my feminine side would say "Oh, no. I'm not worth it. We aren't even going with anyone. It doesn't make any sense."

As I listened to my inner masculine and feminine arguing, I thought, "*Wow, there isn't even anyone here, and I'm having relationship issues.*"

When I considered the masculine protector, I desired a man who looked at me and said, "You look really tired. You've been burning the candle at both ends. You know what? I'm going to draw you a bath. I'm going to take your cell phone, and you are going to take care of you. I'll be in the next room and after your bath, I'm going to give you a nice massage."

Then, I would go through with it. I would turn my phone off. I would go and have a nice bath, then I would get massage oil, and I would rub my body as if I were two people. I would act as if my hand was the hand of a man and have the most wonderful time!

SPONTANEOUS INNER BLISS

The most fascinating thing started happening. As my inner masculine and feminine started loving and honouring each other, I started having spontaneous orgasms in the weirdest places. It's interesting to note that the meaning of "spontaneous" isn't that it happened suddenly. It means that it originated from within!

Once, I was sitting in the library reading a book of poetry. I came across the most beautiful passage. I closed my eyes and just let it soak into me. Suddenly my whole body went into a beautiful bliss state. When I opened my eyes again, I just hoped I hadn't made any weird sounds or anything. Another time, I'd be walking down a busy city street, and I'd feel the sun on my face. I would tip my head back, feel the sun warming my skin, smile, and take a deep breath. With every step, my body would relax a little bit more, and then my whole body would go into a beautiful vibration. It was so incredible!

It's not that spontaneous orgasms are the goal, but they tell us that real happiness is possible within. It is the joy of thinking, "I'd love to do that. Alright, let's do it. I'll make that happen for you." Or "Boy, I'm feeling vulnerable and sad." And then your strong protector comes up and says, "Hey, don't worry. I'll take care of you." Or when you're feeling attacked, your inner protector rises and says "No!" It's so comforting to know that you always have your back.

Inner Balance & Relationships

This inner balance also allows us to fully connect with others. We can't experience healthy masculine and feminine dynamics with another person unless we have our own personal balance.

If we tend to be "ever-masculine", we can't fully unite with another person because we won't be able to connect with their feminine. We won't understand it. We may even be intimidated by it and try to squelch it. Similarly, if we desire to be ever-feminine, it will be very hard to relax in the energy of another person's masculine. If we aren't in a relationship with our inner masculine, we won't be able to discern between healthy and unhealthy masculine in others, so we will always keep a little bit of distance. Plus, if we don't trust our own masculine to show up for us, we won't believe that anyone else will either.

Whatever your inner experience is, you will expect that in the world around you. If your inner masculine is a harsh judge, you'll be fine with bosses, family members, and partners who berate you. If your inner feminine won't receive from your inner masculine, you won't expect to receive from others either.

However, if you have a beautiful balance within, this will be the only dynamic you will expect in the world. If people are overbearing in a relationship, we may discuss this with them to see if they would like to shift that dynamic. If they do, wonderful. If not, we will step aside. If people are needy and have an unhealthy feminine, we may try to help them build up their inner masculine so that they can find balance, but we won't just allow the unhealthy dynamic. We will expect the same balance that we have within, in all of our relationships. It will be the only thing that feels natural.

Androgynous Nature

In the book *Crazy Wisdom of the Yogini*, Daniel Odier talks about the importance of embracing our androgynous nature—that we are both masculine and feminine within. Let's imagine this—that the union of the two makes us completely whole.

We don't need another. We are whole unto ourselves.

Can you imagine what it would be like in relationships if we never needed another person because we are already complete? We could still have whatever relationships we desired, but they would be based on choice. There would be no fear of losing the other person because we are already whole and happy. There would be no more drama in relationships. Everyone would always be acting within choice.

However, as long as we stay disconnected inside, we will continue our need to find and keep our "other half". Due to the separation within, we will always seek it in another person.

FINDING BALANCE WITHIN

The next few chapters take us through many of the dynamics that bring us a wonderful peace within, let us explore all that we want to be, and be excited about everything we create!

Your Personal Journey:

STRENGTHENING THE FEMININE

1. Does your inner feminine know what she wants and desires?
2. Do you listen to your inner feminine desires?
3. Do you take her emotional responses to the world seriously?
4. Does your inner feminine trust your inner masculine's lead?

STRENGTHENING THE MASCULINE

1. Does your inner masculine "show up" for your feminine? Can you count on yourself to always have your back?
2. Do you take your desires seriously? Are they worth giving to yourself?
3. Do you protect yourself from others who may want to harm you or steal your attention and energy?
4. Are you trustworthy to make a good plan for your inner feminine? Or do you make plans that your feminine would never want to carry out?

Chapter 10
Doing & Being

*"You should sit in meditation for 20 minutes a day.
Unless you're too busy, then you should sit for an hour."*
ZEN PROVERB

Masculine is doing, and feminine is being.

This dynamic creates beautiful music within ourselves. Doing is like the musical notes, and Being is the rest in between. Without the rests, musical notes just run together. With the rests, we can savour the melodies, the rise and fall, and the rhythm of the music.

Here, we get to be introspective about what we do in our lives. We can take action and then sit and reflect upon how it went. We can learn from it, grow, and perhaps improve upon our experience the next time or bask in our wonderful success.

Being also lets us sit in contemplation before taking action. I had a calculus professor in university who would give us a seemingly impossible assignment and, seeing our blank and lost faces, would place his palms together in front of his chest and say, "Take this to your place of contemplation and meditate upon it." Then he would smile.

In the beginning, we tend to focus on doing and being separately, as if they are happening sequentially. But eventually, they will exist within each other. While you are resting, you have the awareness of the potential of doing. And within your action, you have the awareness within of being.

Importance of Being

"Doing is never enough if you neglect being."
ECKHART TOLLE

In our world, we do a lot, and we schedule ourselves and our children more and more. I remember car rides when I was a kid, sitting there and just staring out the window. Today, minivans have DVD players for the kids to watch. We are constantly stimulated. We are constantly doing and constantly kept busy.

We must look at how the masculine is born of the feminine in this dynamic—doing is born out of being. If we don't spend enough time being, there will be no gas in the tank. We will burn out. We see this everywhere. And once you are burnt out, you don't have any joy in the doing anymore. The act of being is more important today than ever before.

Historically, we had sayings like, "Idle hands do the devil's handiwork." This may be partially true, in that when we are bored, we can easily distract ourselves with nonsense. It could be doing things we shouldn't be doing or simply wasting our life in front of the TV. It also came out of a time when people had to work very hard, and no one wanted to carry the load of anyone who wasn't doing their share

However, for those who are naturally hard-working, this saying had an unconscious message: "Don't stop working. You mustn't stop to rest. You must always be productive." This is a one-way street to burnout.

We have to have time for just being. When I lived on the farm, it was really important that we took every Sunday off. We needed to rest—to sit on the porch and just look out over the fields (or at each other) for a day.

Today, we must learn and reprogram our minds to "just be." Perhaps this is why we are so drawn to yoga and meditation. When we meditate, it is a big deal to be able to relax. I've taught meditation for a long time, and most people wonder why they can't calm their minds. But we have been trained to believe that there is so much to do. Even in our "downtime", we sit and watch TV, play video games, or scroll on our phones, getting a constant stream of information, advertising, and personalities entering our brains, leading to total mental exhaustion.

So, we practise yoga and meditation. We learn how to breathe deeply which shifts our nervous system out of the "fight or flight" response, and we begin to relax. It is only in this relaxed state that our body starts to rest. Every moment we spend resting, our body heals and becomes stronger.

Going even deeper, being is also an incredible place of peace. When we rest in feminine being, we breathe more deeply. We see the world more clearly. We understand things, and we get a sense of the big picture. Being is a place where we hear wisdom and great ideas.

Importance of Doing

"Talk doesn't cook rice."
CHINESE PROVERB

Due to our human tendency for excessive "doing", in spiritual communities, we will often hear the saying, "You are not a human doing, you are a human being," and it is true. We must take the time to just "be." This is an important antidote to today's busy lifestyle.

However, we are also human doings. Otherwise, why are we here?

For some people, it is their masculine side that is underdeveloped. They are only about being and are very passive in all aspects of their lives. They like to think, analyze, and philosophize about everything, but they take no action. They don't make anything happen in the world. They know everything they are supposed to be doing and thinking. They understand all the great ideas but can't put anything into practice.

If we aren't also doing and making things happen, then our being becomes stagnant. We are not in balance with the world around us.

Sometimes we have a thought or a great idea. If we act on it, that idea now exists in the world as a "something." This sounds incredibly easy and simplistic, but how often do we have ideas and not act on them?

Doing is also part of a healthy emotional feedback loop. If we are feeling sad or depressed, these feelings are meant to inspire us to take action. If we are sad because we are stuck in a relationship that is harmful or essentially dead, in order to truly feel alive, there must be an action that acts on behalf of that feeling. If not, we essentially die inside.

What if you are angry, but you don't do anything about it? The anger consumes you and later will erupt as rage, causing damage and distancing you from others. Action is also key here. Perhaps you need to get to the bottom of what is wrong. Has someone crossed a boundary? Do you feel betrayed? Is the anger a sign that something needs to change?

If we take no action based on our situation, we essentially stop living. But when we take action based on our situation, then rest and reflect, and then take action again, our life becomes very dynamic, interesting, and we feel fully alive.

Your Personal Journey:

STRENGTHENING THE FEMININE

1. How do you enjoy being? Do you meditate, sit by the lake, or go for long walks?
2. Do you have a sense of being all day long?
3. Do you value rest in your day? In your week? What does rest look like? Early to bed? Naps? Meditation?
4. Do you have family or societal training that says that rest is laziness or not acceptable?

Strengthening the Masculine

1. Are you happy making things happen? Do you love taking action?
2. If you struggle to take action, is there a memory that gives a clue as to what created this fear or block?
3. Who do you know who is excellent at getting things done? Why do you think they are so good at it?
4. Do great ideas for what you want to do come from quiet times?

FINDING BALANCE WITHIN

CHAPTER 11

Logic & Intuition

*"It is by logic that we prove,
but by intuition that we discover."*
HENRI POINCARÉ

Logic (masculine) is governed by our left brain and intuition (feminine) by our right brain. There is some truth to the idea that certain people tend to be more left-brained and logical, and others tend to be more right-brained and artistic. However, we can also cultivate the other half of ourselves. We can integrate them so they work together. Just imagine how expansive we would become. What would be possible then?

Listening Within (Feminine)

*"Have the courage to follow your heart and intuition.
They somehow already know
what you truly want to become."*
STEVE JOBS

To connect with our feminine intuition is to hear the wisdom that goes beyond what people are saying or what we've been taught. This is a very different wisdom. It is not just what we have learned from others, books, and training. It is when someone asks us a question, and instead of responding or reacting right away, we

FINDING BALANCE WITHIN

listen within. We scan our inner databanks and then listen to the Universe. We listen inside for an answer.

The question is, how do we hear it every day on a practical level?

When we are looking for an answer, we have built-in mechanisms that guide us in our truth. Unfortunately, through politeness training, expectations of ourselves and others, power struggles, and fears of being alone, we tend to ignore and quiet this wisdom within if it isn't the common or popular opinion.

Years ago, during my healing crisis, I overanalyzed everything. I was always trying to figure out the right way to do things. My teacher, Jim, told me that there are two primary emotions: happy and sad. From there, our brains add in thought patterns creating secondary emotions like frustration, anger, grief, etc.

These primary emotions are our truth about any situation. In order to hear them, we must pay attention to what happens when someone asks us if we want to do something. If our heart lifts, that's a yes (happy). If it drops, that's a no (sad). We may struggle with this truth because we don't want anyone to feel disappointed. But the key is to at least admit to ourselves what our intuition is telling us.

When someone is telling us a story, this same mechanism helps us know if what they are saying is true. As you are listening, your heart will be agreeing, "Yes, yes, yes." Then, they will say something that just doesn't land. It doesn't feel true. This is also our intuition speaking to us. We have no logical reason for knowing that what they are saying isn't quite true, but we simply know. (Note, the person may not be intentionally lying to you. They may be lying to themselves about what is going on or how they feel. But you will still feel the lie… even if they are consciously unaware.)

When we are first learning this, sometimes we still make choices that aren't in alignment with our intuitive truth, which is fine. It is all part of the learning process. The key is to ask ourselves, "Do I trust this yes/no mechanism inside of me? Do I trust that this is divine wisdom that I can follow?"

Divine wisdom doesn't have to be about important things. We are divine and physical beings. This wisdom is for every moment of our day. It is for choosing what to eat, where to go, whether to date that person, how we navigate something with our children, or whether we take this job or that job. Every step is on our soul's journey... all needing guidance.

The Spirit and Thrill of Intuition

This thrill is similar to the exploration of chaos. It is the unknown that draws us. What will come to us that is new and unexpected?

Sometimes intuition simply feels like a hunch. It may not be unexpected at all. You are simply choosing between two options, and one feels right. As we practise listening within and taking action, we soon start to trust our intuition and gut instincts.

Every time we trust them, making decisions becomes easier. We become confident in our intuitive process, and eventually will start to trust it more than our logical minds. Our logical mind simply steps up to support what we know intuitively. This creates incredible conviction and inner strength in the face of adversity while taking positive steps along our life's journey.

The Joy of Logic (Masculine)

Oh, the challenge of figuring something out! To find order within confusion. To create a structure in which we can thrive!

I have a bachelor's degree in mathematics, so I love mental gymnastics. I love looking at a situation, finding the ideal structure to support it, and finding the solution.

Often, when we think of math, we think of addition and multiplication. However, mathematics is so much more than that. It is actually a philosophy. It is the marriage of intuition and logic. It is the process of trying to map the Universe in the simplest format—numbers.

When you picture a mathematician standing in front of a blackboard covered with equations, what are they doing? Thinking. Sometimes they are thinking logistically, trying to see what is wrong with the equations on the board. If they come to a stalemate, they must wonder if their assumptions are correct. Perhaps they aren't looking at the problem properly.

So, they relax their left brain and allow their right brain to wander. What else is possible? What am I not seeing? How else could we look at this? How else could it make sense?

Then they have a Eureka moment! In floods the math brain again. Yes! We can apply this theorem to that! Yes, of course, we missed the step here in the logic! Brilliant!

BEING OF SOBER MIND

Mr. Spock is a well-known Vulcan character from Star Trek. The Vulcans were renowned for their logical and unemotional minds. Having a bit of Vulcan inside of us can be very valuable.

Logic comes from a sober mind. This sobriety is not being drunk on emotions, hope, or the need to make others happy. A sober mind is free to look directly at a problem and see it with a kind of Vulcan clarity.

Although this kind of clarity is void of emotion, it is incredibly valuable—especially when paired with intuition. Often, our intuition asks us to do things that are outside the box and hard to understand. Logic may not have the answers as to why, but a sober mind will help us to see the possible benefits and downfalls and help us to make a solid decision that we can feel good about.

Our Brains Working Together

There are times when we are only using one side of our brains. Perhaps, we are doing accounting, and our left, masculine, logical side is happily counting, sorting, and solving problems. In this case,

LOGIC & INTUITION

the bliss of union comes from applying your logic and structure to the "chaos" in the books before you and sorting it out.

In the same way, if a creative mind is given a structure to work within, then you will be in bliss as you embrace being in full flow. Let's say you are a home decorator. Once you understand the parameters, scope, and limitations of the job, then your creativity can flow.

Einstein is one of my favourite role models. He was not only fully balanced between his left and right brains, but his brains were also beautifully integrated. He had an incredible, mathematical, scientific mind but he also stopped and pondered the Universe. He thought about what else was possible. He pondered things that had never been thought of before. He didn't think within the box. He liked to delete the box of current theories and then go beyond.

When Einstein died, they wanted to study his brain. What did a brain like his look like? How was it different from others?

First, we must understand our brains. When we are born, our brain is mostly gray matter—raw neurons. As we learn and develop, a white myelin sheath forms around the gray matter, and it becomes white matter. This is called becoming myelinated. As soon as you learn something, like tying your shoes, you now have this superhighway of white matter in that area of the brain, and the task becomes effortless.

Both of the hemispheres of Einstein's brain were heavily myelinated—the left side due to his mathematical, scientific and logical mind, and the right side due to his ponderings about what was possible in the world, imagined mystery, and thought beyond the regular constructs. Plus, he played music and was very creative.

In between the left and right hemispheres is a band of nerves called the corpus callosum where communication flows between the two sides. The more connected our left and right brains are, the more myelinated it is. Well, Einstein's corpus callosum was completely white matter. It was as if the left and the right side were fused.

This is actually our goal. We don't need to walk around thinking, "Okay, well, now I'm going to be logical. And now, I'm going to be intuitive." Ideally, it all just flows together and becomes seamless.

To Einstein, he wouldn't have to distinguish between what was logical and what was intuitive. It all just blended together into a whole. This is where it is beautiful. It is not that the left brain is better than the right brain or that artists rule the world and mathematicians don't. They are meant to be connected, and to honour the brilliance of both.

This is perhaps where the genius lies within all of us.

Your Personal Journey:

Strengthening the Feminine

1. How do you hear your intuition? Is it in meditation or prayer? Sitting by the ocean? Discussing with friends?
2. Do you trust what you hear inside as divine wisdom?
3. Do you have friends who are intuitive and who you could learn more from? How do they navigate? How do they trust what they hear inside?
4. If logic is your go-to, how could you bring more intuition into the game?

Strengthening the Masculine

1. Are you able to access your sober mind? Can meditation help to calm your mind so that you can see with Vulcan clarity?
2. Do you have friends who are very logical and could help you develop this side of yourself?
3. If intuition is your go-to, how could you bring more logic into your world?
4. How do you access your logical mind? Physical activity? Meditation? Journaling?

Chapter 12

Inspiration & Manifestation

*"Life is either a daring adventure
or nothing at all."*
HELEN KELLER

Living the Life We Were Born to Live

This is the dynamic of being inspired (feminine) and then manifesting our idea (masculine). It is an artist seeing a vision in their mind and painting it. They are taking what they see inside and putting it out into the world.

Inspiration, wisdom, and listening within for guidance are all feminine because they are ways that we receive information. We are receiving information from the Universe, the situation, and our highest self.

Their partner is manifestation. We can have all the greatest ideas in the world. We can receive whatever guidance we want, but if we don't do anything with it and bring it into the physical world, it is of no earthly good. This is where we just talk and tell ourselves things. We make lists which make us feel like we have done things, even though we sometimes never complete the lists.

The deeper importance of this dynamic is that it allows us to live the life that we are born to live. We get to truly listen to who *we* are, what *we* want out of life, what *we* believe in, and then bring that into the world. It is about having the freedom and the courage to manifest what we see and feel inside.

It could be the job we take, who we marry, what we look like, or what we do in our spare time. It is literally bringing ourselves out into the world.

In theory, this shouldn't be so difficult, and I don't think it always will be. I think that down the road it will be natural, and there are a lot of people who do this already, but it isn't the norm. We tend to be very outwardly focused on what we need to do and what we should be doing. We are ruled by shoulds a lot. It is a quite new idea that we could all live this way—excited, at peace, and creating our lives.

Existentially, when we manifest our dreams, we feel like we matter and that we are alive with some purpose. We are happy. We are engaged. We are optimistic. We feel fully alive.

It also strengthens the masculine and feminine within us and how we act with others. When I feel confident that I will manifest whatever I feel called to do, my masculine is strengthened, and not just in this dynamic, it is strengthened in all dynamics. Similarly, if I know that I can listen and trust what I hear within and receive it, that will strengthen my feminine in all interactions.

Feminine Inspiration

Feminine inspiration comes from listening within. It is funny how uncommon this is, considering it is the only way we will manifest the life that is unique to us. Of course, being unique has not always been seen as a good thing. In books and movies, there is often the character of the outlier—that crazy person who lives at the edge of town and doesn't follow any of the rules. They do unexpected things, they do things on the wrong days of the week, they don't attend town meetings, and they don't dress properly.

Our myths are interesting because they tell us a lot about where our belief systems come from. For example, in this outlier story, we learn to demonize the people who look different and who act differently. So, why would we risk listening within? What if we hear something that is different from the crowd? What if we hear a call that would make us stand out and potentially become an outlier?

The idea of listening within and manifesting what we feel called to do is no small thing. It is important for our soul's path because we often don't realize how much we have conformed in the past and held our true selves back. Most of us have been forced into a kind of robotic, very tamed life.

The ability to listen within is a new skill. As children, we learned that we have to listen to our parents. Then we go to school, and we are taught to give the right answer to get a good mark or to be successful. There are always exceptions, but by and large, we don't strengthen the muscle that seeks the answer within. Instead, we strengthen the muscle that helps us to look around to see what would be acceptable and what would appear to be a success to others, whether we internally feel it or not.

However, we are humans. We are meant to do interesting things and manifest our dreams. So, it is important to figure out how to hear that inspiration, trust it, and then summon the courage and excitement to take action.

Manifestation

Manifestation is born out of inspiration. The stronger the inspiration, the easier it is to trust it, manifest it, and create it. It is our masculine that puts on our running shoes and goes running. Our masculine puts out a yoga mat and does the yoga. It is our masculine that launches the new business, takes painting classes, and decides to learn Spanish.

FINDING BALANCE WITHIN

This is a big deal because this is what makes us feel alive. It makes us feel like we actually exist on the planet. I had an idea, and I made it happen. Another idea appeared, and I did that. This is when the masculine-feminine dances together. We feel alive. We feel like we matter. We have joyful confidence in life.

It doesn't even matter if what we did worked out. This isn't about success. We aren't counting our successes or stockpiling great stories of inspiration and manifestation. That is not the point. The point is enjoying the energy of the dance. The point is, "I have this great idea. I tried it. Wow, that was really entertaining. Didn't quite work out the way I thought, but what an amazing experience it was to manifest this idea inside of me."

It is like getting up to do a morning spiritual or exercise practice. When we do it, we feel like a million bucks all day. But so often, five seconds before getting up, we have to decide to let our masculine step in and roll out our yoga mat or tie up our running shoes. One voice might say, "I feel tired. I don't want to." But another voice says, "Come on. Let's do it!"

Manifestation is the feeling of something wanting to be born. You can feel the moment of conception—the idea appearing inside. You start to feel the seed growing. Even though it may not be obvious to others, and there is no visible "baby bump," you can feel the life inside of you starting to grow. The idea continues to ferment, steep, and brew within. Maybe you talk to your friends about it. Maybe you do some market research to see if it's a good idea. Maybe you journal and dream about it on paper.

Manifestation is the day of birth. This is when the idea is no longer inside. It is now manifest in the world. It could be a new business, a piece of art, a song, a book, learning a new language, or an important conversation with a loved one. This is the real excitement in life!

Potential Struggles with Manifestation

FEAR OF JUDGEMENT

One of the things that blocks us from creating and manifesting is that we might not be able to explain what we're doing to others. It might be new, outside of the norm, or outside of the accepted practice. We are so afraid of the judgement of others. We are so afraid that they are going to think what we did was wrong, foolish, or that we aren't great at it.

A lot of this starts in school. We learned that only the best people do certain things, and everyone else is a spectator. The best athletes play sports, and the rest of us watch. The best musicians play concerts and we all listen. The best artists create, and everyone else buys their paintings.

I once asked a friend of mine if she played the guitar. She said, "Oh yes, very badly," and just smiled. She loved playing the guitar but had no intention of being "good" at it. She knew she didn't want to spend the hours needed in order to master it. That wasn't why she was doing it. She just loved to play the guitar.

I was asking her because I wanted to learn to play the guitar. I wanted to be able to play around the campfire and sing songs with my family and the kids. So, I decided to just learn how to strum and make a few chords. I never even learned all the chords, and if I was playing a song and I didn't know the chord, I would just stop playing until we passed it. It was so much fun!

There is a real joy in getting to do something "badly," without judgement, and saying, "I just want to play."

Back in 1999, during my healing crisis, my teacher knew that I was struggling with the judgement of others. I thought about what others would think all day long. One day, he asked me to do a Taoist practice called monkey medicine. Basically, I had to go into a room by myself, take off all my clothes, and jump around like a monkey. I had to make sounds like a monkey, scratching myself and jumping all over the room.

The shocker was that I couldn't do it. I could not act like a monkey all by myself in a room. It was a very potent lesson. I'd been telling myself that I was afraid of what *other* people thought, but it actually had nothing to do with what *other* people thought. It was all me.

This internal judgement is a huge part of our fears in manifestation.

BEING A SPECTATOR

The idea of manifesting something ourselves might also seem like a foreign concept because we are often trained to be spectators, as previously mentioned, in school.

Look at how we have been wired to watch TV. We pay other people a lot of money to play sports. We watch documentaries about people diving in the Caribbean. We watch other people follow their dreams, renovate their houses, and live their own lives. We literally have become a world of spectators.

To then imagine that we could do something ourselves might seem very new. The shift from spectator to participant or creator is definitely a big one.

FEAR OF FAILURE

I love reading about entrepreneurs — especially famous ones — who have "failed" a lot. We tend to only hear about the ones who "made it." We have no insight at all into all the ventures that didn't work.

The key with these entrepreneurs, these huge manifesters, is that their joy is in the creative process. For example, Sir Richard Branson created Virgin Airlines, Virgin Records, Virgin Telecom, and countless other companies. For all the ventures you've heard about, he has just as many failed attempts. He just loves manifesting. He loves having a great idea and then letting his masculine do the math and figure out the plan. It is a great way to feel alive.

INSPIRATION & MANIFESTATION

The thrill is in the excitement. However, if manifesting is new to us, we easily misinterpret excitement as fear. We think, "What if it fails? What if it works? What if it doesn't?"

But this is natural. This is how we should feel. If you are at the top of a mountain on a BMX bike, you can see the rocky terrain that you have to navigate. Excitement builds inside of you because you have to focus. You don't know what's going to happen. That's the point. You have to be single-minded. You get to respond in each moment. That is excitement. That is truly being alive.

We have been in the safe spectator role for so long that we have forgotten what this excitement feels like. We have forgotten what the feeling of success versus failure feels like. What if it succeeds? What if it is a bust? If it was fun, that's all that matters. It is not about the end result. It is about the whole—the possible destination, the journey, and every experience in between.

Your Personal Journey:

STRENGTHENING THE FEMININE

1. What is something that you would love to manifest in your life?
2. How do you hear inspiration? In the bath, journaling, on a run, at random times?
3. Was there a time in your life when you stopped listening within for insight and inspiration? Why did you stop? Can you bring it back?
4. Do you trust your inspiration as something that wants to be manifested?

STRENGTHENING THE MASCULINE

1. What have you created in the past that worked out great?
2. What fears stand in the way of creating what you desire in your life? Where do they come from?

FINDING BALANCE WITHIN

3. What would it take to get you out of the stands and really participate in life?
4. Who do you know that is excellent at manifesting? What can you learn from their process?

SECTION IV

Sexual Intimacy & Divine Union

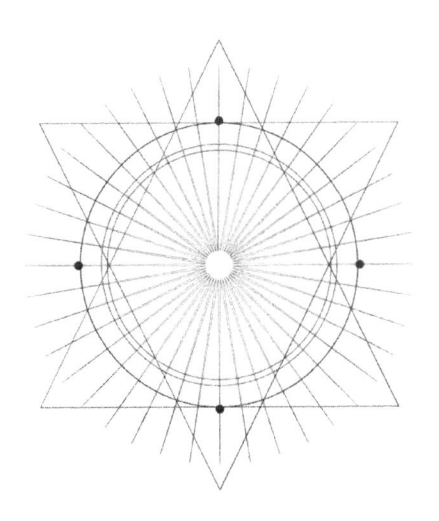

Chapter 13

Romantic Relationships

*"He bowed to enter his cart. He lit a candle.
He was too tall for the low ceiling, but she was smaller and
could stand straight. The candles made huge shadows.*

*His bed was open, merely a blanket thrown back.
His clothes were strewn around. There were two guitars.
He took one up and began to play, sitting among his clothes.*

*Hilda had the feeling that she was dreaming, that she must keep
her eyes on his bare arms, on his throat showing through his
open shirt so that he would feel what she felt—the same
magnetism.*

*At the same moment that she felt she was falling into darkness
into his golden-brown feet, he fell towards her and covered her
with kisses, very hot, quick kisses, into which his breath passed.
He kissed her behind her ears, on her eyelids,
her throat, her shoulders.*

*She was blinded, deafened, made senseless.
Every kiss, like a gulp of wine, added to the warmth of her body."*
LITTLE BIRDS by ANAÏS NIN

The Magic of Romance

The passion of eros sparks something inside of us fueling this magnetism like nothing else. Therefore, this is where we get to play in the polarity through which our energy wants to flow the most.

In all other aspects of our lives, we play as whole beings—fully balanced in the masculine and feminine. But in romance, there is a desire for a different depth of union. It is partly sex, partly love, and partly the desire to completely merge with another person.

It is interesting how it can't be with just anyone. There is something specific about the people for whom we have erotic desire. Have we known each other before? Are we returning to a previously experienced united state of bliss? Are we meant for each other? Is there something more going on than we know?

It's hard to say, but an exploration of the polarities is the most exciting way to find out.

My Discovery of Tantra

There are many ways to make love and show love for each other. In this section, it is tantric, intimate connection that we are talking about.

I was married to a wonderful man for twenty years. Throughout that time, there was love, support, and lots of great sex. For all intents and purposes, we had a wonderful marriage, but something inside of me was saying, "There's more possible." I had a sense that there was a deeper kind of intimacy. Although our sex life was full of kindness, orgasms, and great kissing, I knew that we were somehow just scratching the surface when it came to what was possible in sexual intimacy.

This is when I discovered Tantra, and I knew that it held the keys to what I was seeking. If you would like to dive deeper into Tantra, please check out my book: *Tantric Intimacy: Discover the Magic of True Connection.*

ROMANTIC RELATIONSHIPS

Tantra is a spiritual path that asks us to look at life very differently. Tantra sees every one of us as fully divine and physical beings. Tantra sees every moment of our life as an opportunity to experience depth and bliss.

One of the beautiful things about knowing that we are both divine and physical is that it becomes easier to drop our guards because our fears disappear. We easily see our lover as the divine person they are. We slow down and notice subtleties of gaze, presence, and touch.

This slowing down process in intimacy allows us the time to connect energetically, emotionally, and physically. We are no longer just having sex. We are exploring the possibility of merging with another person. We are no longer just desiring an orgasm. We are seeking orgasmic bliss.

How do we achieve this orgasmic bliss? By deeply connecting and returning to oneness.

How do we do that? Through the total merging of the polarities to create a new whole.

Joys of Polarity

In many sexual encounters, we can often find ourselves both acting in the masculine. I do this, then she does this. He does this, then I do that. Everyone is doing something to the other. It is more like a tennis match—a masculine-masculine experience.

However, when we polarize into the masculine and feminine, we create a circuit of energy. The more the masculine gives, the more the feminine opens. The more the feminine opens, the more the masculine is energized to give. As this continues, the energy builds and builds, getting bigger and bigger and stronger and stronger. Once the energy starts to flow, we barely care about or notice what we are doing. We are just playing in the energy. It is exciting and pleasurable but not in the "chasing the orgasm" way. It is an entirely different game.

So, what exactly does it mean to be masculine in intimacy? It means that you love to pursue your partner and initiate lovemaking. You love giving, touching, caressing, and kissing them. You love to be the stillness to their chaos and wildness. In intimacy involving a *vajra* (Sanskrit word for penis meaning "thunderbolt"), this means being able to control your ejaculation so that your partner can go into wild waves of orgasmic bliss for as long as desired.

Being feminine in intimacy means that you want to explore your wildness. You want to fully open yourself to your partner. You want to open yourself as the Earth opens herself to the rain. As you openly receive, your nervous system relaxes and can carry orgasmic energy through you. As both of your energy bodies start to merge, you then get to flow in this river of pleasure together.

Let's imagine you are receiving a massage. You are in full receptive mode, and the giver is in full giving mode. There is joy in each person's experience. The giver can 100% focus on reading their partner, listen to their intuition, and give whatever the receiver needs in each moment. Similarly, the receiver can fully surrender and completely lose themselves in the experience. The more the receiver relaxes and trusts, the more the giver can give and feels confident to give. Both are able to surrender in their own way, energy flows freely between them, and something truly magical happens.

However, let's instead say that you are each sitting on opposite ends of the couch and massaging each other's feet. You are both being masculine and feminine at the same time. You can really only give 50% of yourself to receiving the foot massage and 50% to giving the foot massage. However, if your partner touches a particularly wonderful spot on your foot, you will stop massaging for a moment, take a deep breath, and fully receive this pleasure. We will slip into 100% polarity to experience this total bliss.

Once the pleasurable experience has passed, you might go back into the neutral place of giving and receiving at the same time. This can be a kind and loving experience, but it doesn't allow us the depth of pleasure and bliss that full polarization brings.

Choosing Our Preferred Polarity

We must first ask ourselves whether we prefer to be in the feminine or the masculine polarity. Would we like to explore the chaos, mystery, and receiving of the feminine? Or would we prefer to strengthen the power, structure, and giving of the masculine? This is regardless of gender or orientation. It is about finding the energy polarity that grows and expands us.

For example, most heterosexual women are strengthened by being in the feminine, learning to receive, and exploring their vulnerability. They expand when able to let go completely. It empowers them, and it makes them deeper and stronger. Similarly, it is very empowering for heterosexual men to be the structure, strength, and giving energy in the passion energy circuit.

In same-sex couples and other wonderful combinations, each partner will have a tendency toward a certain polarity. One partner will be empowered and strengthened in the masculine role and the other partner will love to receive and play in the wild feminine.

(If you don't desire polarization or are asexual, you may fall into one of the other kinds of relationships that we discussed in Chapter 3, and this exploration of polarized, romantic play doesn't apply to your situation.)

Why We Default to the Polarity That Doesn't Strengthen Us

This is where a very specific argument can arise. It could be heterosexual women saying, "No way! I like being in the masculine!" and the men saying, "Why do I have to be in the masculine? I want to receive and be pursued." We will explore this in the heterosexual pattern, but it applies to all other orientations as well.

Let's say you are a heterosexual man who would love to be considered the masculine in the relationship. However, you were raised in a home where flying under the radar meant safety, or if you stuck your neck out and tried something different, you would be judged. Choosing to be in the masculine becomes a scary idea and something to be avoided. You may easily get into the habit of taking (and enjoying) the backseat in relationships. If someone else is driving, then you can't be judged or get into trouble.

This man will often be attracted to a woman who embodies the masculine—planning and doing everything. She might have realized early on in life that if she doesn't do it, it isn't going to get done. If she's not in control, she will be stepped on or ignored. In a similar way, she will be attracted to a man who doesn't get in her way and is easily swayed by her opinion.

Although the woman seems to be in the masculine and the man seems to be in the feminine, they actually aren't because how they act doesn't lead to union. They are still disconnected. She is simply in control, and he is going along with her. There is no giving-receiving, structure-chaos, protector-vulnerable, or pursuer-pursuit going on between them. She is in control (not masculine) and he is just passive (not feminine).

Deep down, many of these men would love to be in the masculine. The problem is that they don't want to be the stereotypical controlling masculine they've experienced in the past. Similarly, many women secretly desire to be in their full feminine (hence the blockbuster sales of the book *Fifty Shades of Grey* where the heroine is completely dominated by her BDSM lover. Most of the readers were women and were not into BDSM of any kind. However, they secretly craved that powerful masculine-feminine dynamic where they got to be the willing feminine!).

This is similar in same-sex couples. Years ago, there was a gay man who took my tantra course. Once he learned about this masculine and feminine dynamic, he had an "aha" moment about why his relationships often didn't work if both partners were actually "femmes"—preferring the feminine polarity or "bottom." In order to be sexually intimate, one of them would have to shift polarity into the masculine (or be a "top"). They shifted polarity because they were attracted to each other and wanted to be intimate. But deep down, they didn't want to be in the masculine. It wasn't the polarity that was expansive for them. Once this shift became the norm in the relationship, passive-aggressive arguments would start to rise. The one who had to switch wasn't actually happy with their sacrifice but wasn't able to explain why.

He said that the most effortless relationships were when he was with someone who was a natural masculine because he was a natural feminine. They were the most dynamic and fun because both partners got to grow and expand in the ways that felt most natural and exciting for them.

The Polarity Continuum

Even if we prefer one polarity in intimate relationships, it isn't 100% of the time. Maybe 70% of the time you like being in the masculine and 30% in the feminine. Maybe 20% of the time you like to be in the masculine and 80% in the feminine.

It's important that this has nothing to do with how we act in the rest of our life. We must be able to take either polarity throughout our regular days depending on the situation. Here, we are just talking about intimate romantic relationships where a more magical magnetism is possible.

Personally, I love being the feminine in romantic relationships. My preference would be to be 90% in the feminine and 10% in the masculine. So, the most dynamic and fun relationships for me are when I'm with someone who loves to be the opposite — 90% in the masculine and 10% in the feminine.

Now imagine if I was in a relationship where the other person wanted to be 60% in the masculine and 40% in the feminine. You can imagine that we would be happy in our romantic relationship some of the time. However, neither of us would be fully satisfied in the long run because I wouldn't want to be in the masculine often enough to make them happy and vice versa.

Your Personal Journey:

1. What is your preference in intimacy? Masculine or feminine?
2. What would your ideal ratio be? What percentage masculine to feminine? 90/10, 70/30, 50/50, 80/20?
3. Do you tend to be in the flipped polarity in relationships? Do you tend to be controlling when you'd prefer to be in the feminine? Or do you take a back seat when you'd actually rather be in the masculine? Where do you think this comes from?
4. How have your relationships looked according to this pairing? Have certain relationships been easier because you each desired the opposite polarity? Have there been others where you both were in the same polarity? What were those like?

Chapter 14
The Passion of Pursuit

My friend was in a super passionate relationship. Her partner would come home and make dinner, and they would dance in the kitchen. They would have amazing sex and talk long into the night. It was everything she ever wanted.

Then, bit by bit, that started to disappear. He began to play more video games and didn't want to sit and chat as much. Things became very comfortable, easy, and relaxed, and besides a little sex before sleep, he never seemed to want to do anything with her anymore.

So, she bought sexy lingerie. She planned fun things for them to do. When that didn't work, she assumed that maybe she had done or said something wrong and spent serious time looking inwards. Then, she became very busy with life and financial issues and let her concerns about their relationship sit on the back burner.

After a couple of years, she asked him what happened. "It just feels like you don't put any effort in anymore. Like you don't care. Like you're not attracted to me."

He just looked at her point blank and said, "Why run to catch a bus you've already caught?"

Although my friend's partner was pretty blunt, this has been a prevailing belief in our society—that passion all comes at the beginning. That there is a honeymoon period. That there is the initial excitement, and then you relax into something much easier and more comfortable. And there is some truth in that. Normally, we can fall into a much more relaxed relationship as we get to know each other and as we feel more comfortable in that love.

However, we need to have passion if we want to have a dynamic relationship. If we want to have that excitement, joy, and magnetism, then we need to keep fuelling that fire. However, this art of pursuit has been lost in our society. There are always exceptions where people are always in pursuit of each other, and they keep their relationship alive and strong, but it has not been the norm.

What if, instead, it was normal for our connection to deepen over time? What if every step took us on a new adventure together? What if romance got more exciting over the years and our passion continued to grow and grow?

The Energy of Pursuit

Note: For the rest of the book, due to the unwieldiness of saying "the partner who prefers the feminine," I may say her *or* she. *If it is this wider font, then I am referring to the feminine partner regardless of gender. Similarly, I may say* him *or* he, *referring to the masculine partner regardless of gender.*

Pursuit activates the primal part of the masculine. It is the hunter, that excited primal being that says, "Yes, I'm alive! I know what I love, I know what I want, and I'm going for it!" Because this strengthens the masculine partner, there is more magnetism between the couple. This strong magnetic force is felt as live vibrational energy. The relationship is alive and well.

In all aspects of our lives, pursuit isn't just about getting something you want. It is about discovery. It is about discovering the mystery of the feminine—either within ourselves or in another. The feminine is by nature mysterious. There is something magical about the energy of pursuit—the adventure of the unknown, sailing ships to explore uncharted seas, and finding out what else is possible in this infinite life.

Pursuit is the excitement of exploring new aspects of life, personal dreams, and intimacy. For those who desire dynamic and passionate relationships, pursuit is the primary movement of all excitement.

Pursuit in Intimacy

In romantic relationships, this is a dynamic where we definitely want to explore our preferred polarity. The thrill is always the masculine energy pursuing the mysterious feminine. This could be planning date nights, bringing home flowers, giving a massage, or anything that is unnecessary in day-to-day life, but makes the feminine know that they are desired. It is doing things for our partner that they would love and that we would love to do for them. It is like imagining every day is your first date, and you really want to make this person feel special.

First, we have to get to know our lover well enough to know what they would like. Is it going out for dinner? Is it dancing? Is it music? Is it candles? Is it a massage? What is it that they really love?

The next question is for the masculine partner. What do you love to do? How do you love to pursue someone? Is it planning a beautiful meal out? Is it making a meal in? Is it setting up a beautiful romantic evening or planning a weekend away? What is it that you love to do? How do these things overlap with how your partner would love to be pursued?

Initiating Intimacy

Initiating intimacy is a big part of this masculine polarity. When the masculine pursues sexually, something wakes up in their partner. Something deep within is stimulated as they decide whether or not to surrender to this pursuit.

There may be times when the feminine partner initiates. Sometimes their polarities will remain flipped for lovemaking, which can be very exciting. Other times, the feminine may initiate, and then their partner happily takes over the masculine role. But there is something extra special when the person who prefers the masculine initiates and continues in that role. It is the powerful masculine energy that flows through them that is important. They have an endless well of energy for them to pour into the feminine. When that energy is activated, it is like a raging river flowing into you. The magnetism is stronger. The energy flows effortlessly. The lovemaking flows easily, naturally, and is so exciting.

Being Pursued

I once had a vision where I was in a temple surrounded by other goddesses. I was sitting on the floor happily brushing my hair. My hand holding the brush was my masculine, and my hair and head were the feminine, receiving this wonderful experience. My masculine loved brushing my hair, and my feminine was in her glory. I sat there in total bliss, in total union with myself.

Then, a man came along and placed his hand gently on my brush indicating that he wanted to take over brushing my hair. I closed my eyes to register this new energy and realized that this would feel wonderful. I released my brush to him and then allowed myself to feel this new experience. As I felt the brush massaging my head, I began to relax and polarize into the full feminine. As I relaxed, he knelt down to wrap his arm around my shoulder while he continued brushing. Bit by bit, I allowed him to hold me as I released further into the experience. Eventually, we blended into a beautiful oneness—even more wonderful than my previous state.

Being pursued in the feminine is not an action. It isn't about wearing certain clothes and making sure people notice you. We must remember the difference between the masculine and feminine. The masculine is doing, the action, and the energy. The feminine is being. Until a masculine draws us out of ourselves, we exist in wholeness.

Once pursuit begins, something happens within the feminine. She begins to fill with anticipation. Her desire for love and connection expands with colours and loving energy. As she fully polarizes into the feminine, she becomes like a vacuum—a fully negative pole. As the masculine continues to pursue, he is pulled in magnetically seemingly against his will. She continues to expand and expand, releasing herself to this new experience.

Being pursued by someone you desire is very exciting, but how do we stay content within ourselves before that happens? How do we resist shifting into the masculine and pursuing someone we are interested in?

BEING WHOLE & COMPLETE

Wholeness is the key to being in the feminine. Ideally, every person is always in blissful wholeness. Whether we are in a relationship or not is irrelevant to our happiness. If we choose to be in a relationship, that's great. If not, also wonderful!

Of course, this hasn't been the norm for a long time. Sometimes we have biological clocks ticking that say we must find a mate to have children. Or maybe we struggle with self-worth and need the special attention of another to prove to us that we are lovable or to fill in the love we didn't receive as children. Most often, we are taught through our families and Hollywood that there is no excitement like the excitement of romance and marriage. All of these things can leave us in a perpetual state of high alert and wanting.

Of course, there is nothing wrong with desiring a partner or lover. Human touch and affection are important aspects of being human that truly nourish us. The key here is this desire doesn't rule us. If someone doesn't pursue us, we are not heartbroken or depressed about it.

When we are whole, we are happy one way or another. This is the only state of being where we can actually be pursued. If we feel desperation for someone, we will likely pursue them, and be in the masculine. Sometimes this works out great because they just needed to know that you liked them, too. Sometimes they still don't desire you which is why they never pursued you in the first place. Other times, they accept your pursuit and a relationship ensues. But it is only alive while you are in the masculine. We will talk more about that later in the "Bait and Switch" section.

The biggest key here is that we have an exciting life on our own. When we are fully engaged in our passions and interests and expanding in all aspects of our lives, we aren't just "waiting around" for someone to pursue us. We are out painting, riding horses, writing books, dancing, and swimming in the sea. We are having fun with our friends and learning Spanish.

This is what allows us to be happily pursued by the masculine. We are content. If they come to brush our hair, wonderful. If not, also wonderful. It's all good.

Cultural Differences

Pursuit can appear differently in different cultures. I am obviously using a wide paintbrush because nothing applies to everyone in any culture. But regardless, some interesting dynamics can be observed for the sake of seeing different patterns.

There are cultures like the Spanish and Italian that are known to be very passionate. There is a passion in the men, and pursuing the feminine is easy for them. There is no question that they will pursue. In response, the women will easily say, "Oh wonderful," or "No, I'm not interested" in which case the men say, "Okay, I will go." In passionate countries, the pursuit is easier, saying no is easier, and, ideally, no one takes it personally.

Then there are other cultures (like Canada where I live) where pursuit and passion are not the norm. If the masculine says, "I am interested in you." and the feminine person says, "Sorry, I'm not interested in you", the masculine often feels and acts rejected. This causes the feminine to have a harder time saying no in the future because they don't want to hurt anyone's feelings.

I'd like to share two examples with you.

When my daughter was seventeen, she went to Finland on a Rotary exchange. For one year, she went to school with the Finnish kids. In Finland, there's a cultural gender equality where the masculine seldom pursues the feminine. It's almost an insult if they do because everyone expects to be treated the same.

Well, she was friends with another exchange student from Mexico who was having a very hard time with this. The Finnish boys were driving her crazy. She was attracted to some of them, but they never pursued her. In her culture, women never pursued men. Later, she found out that the Finnish boys might have asked her out after a couple of years of knowing her. In the meantime, she just kept asking my daughter, "What's wrong with these guys?!" The cultures totally clashed. She was waiting for this amazing, romantic, passionate polarity, and it wasn't going to happen.

Another time, I was in Portugal at a dance retreat where we explored African dances like Kizomba with teachers who had come up from Angola to teach us. It was so amazing! One evening, we discussed the challenges of nightclubs where they danced these dances in Europe.

It was often a challenge when the African men would dance with some European women. The women would often get angry because they felt like the men were too forward. They always seemed to be going too far. Kizomba, for example, can be a very sensual dance. You begin with a decent frame, and as the dance progresses, the men can bring the woman closer and closer until the bodies are pressing up against each other. It can be very connected and intimate.

This was a massive misunderstanding between the cultures. In Africa, the men knew that the women would dictate how wide their frame was and how close they could come. It was up to the woman, the one being pursued, to set the boundaries. It was the woman who would say, "Oh, this is as far as we are going to go. I'll let you know when you can come closer." The women never pursued the men, but they would give guidance as to how far the men could go because the men were naturally in pursuit mode. They were easily in that positive magnetism.

However, when dancing in Europe, these magnetically positive men were getting into all kinds of trouble. The women felt like they were being sexually harassed, and the men had no idea what they were talking about. They were just dancing. However, many of the European women hadn't been trained to dictate their boundaries in this way. They had been raised in a more patriarchal culture where you didn't question the men and you didn't want to hurt their feelings. You also didn't want to be perceived as anything but fun and easy to get along with. And so, while dancing, the African men would pull the European women in close, and the women wouldn't say anything, quietly getting uncomfortable, angrier and offended, and the men had no idea what was wrong.

I remember when I first went to Italy, a friend of mine said, "Well, whatever you do, Katrina, if a man comes on to you, he might be wanting dinner, to get married, or to just have sex. Whatever you do, just be totally honest."

They literally had to tell me to be honest! They had to tell me to ignore my normal man-pleasing tendency of coddling their egos and holding back my thoughts. They had to tell me that these men and their culture of pursuing women were different, and I had to act more like an Italian woman and less like a Canadian one.

Then there are places in the world where the unhealthy patriarchy is still very strong. Men do pursue, but not in a way in which the women want to be pursued. It feels lecherous and controlling. There is a sense that men can do anything they want, and women are just sexual objects to be admired or attained.

In all situations, communication is key. If we are from different cultures, then we need to explain where we are coming from. We need to be clear about what we desire and honour our truth. Then, we can choose to play together or go our separate ways.

Challenges in Pursuit

LACK OF PURSUIT

I've worked with many couples where the masculine partner does not pursue the feminine and all passion in the relationship dries up. Both people assume that this is normal—that the fire always goes out of a relationship eventually. They and the relationship become like an arid desert.

Sometimes, the man wasn't the romantic[3] type to begin with and, after the initial excitement of dating, he just relaxed back into what he truly wanted—a comfortable life without having to put effort into a relationship. Often, the women took this personally. They felt that the lack of pursuit had something to do with their attractiveness and desirability.

Many of the women had been with their husbands since their early 20s. This was the only serious relationship they had ever had, and because they were so attached to their husband, how he felt about them really mattered. As the passion waned (or never existed), they often made excuses to themselves and others, saying that their husband was just really tired from working so hard. Maybe he had a difficult upbringing, and they were just being understanding as to why he wasn't as openly loving as they wished.

Sometimes, the wives would get angry and emotional. Some even got mean and sarcastic, desperately trying to wake their partner up. More often, they just quietly disappeared and let the dream of that romantic relationship die inside. Bit by bit, their sexual passion waned. No matter how sensual they might once have felt, when it was ignored by their partner, there was just no point in feeling that way anymore.

They often noticed this early in the relationship, but once children came into the picture, the woman could focus her love and attention

---

[3] Romantic = desiring the passion of the masculine and feminine dance

on them. The husband was off the hook while his wife dove into the world of motherhood.

By the time they came to me for help, the children had moved out, and it was just the two of them. Sometimes, the husband would reach out to me hoping that tantra could help his wife desire sex again. Sometimes the woman would reach out hoping that tantra could help her husband become interested in her again. But by that time, there was no spark left. The arid desert wasn't just empty. It was filled with resentment, disappointment, and a lot of hurt feelings.

Many of these couples divorced a few years later. The women realized that they really did want romance, pursuit, and flowers, and their husbands simply didn't. Others stayed together out of convenience and ease and let go of their desire for pursuit or romance.

The key is to be aware of your potential partner from the beginning. If you desire romance and pursuit, honestly observe if your masculine partner wants this too. If they don't make any moves to pursue you while you're dating, they won't once you're in a committed relationship. So, romance might not be part of this relationship if you go forward with it.

Of course, there are those who practise "love-bombing" while dating like our friend in the story and then things slowly go dry. If this happens, the key is constant communication with each other and honesty with ourselves as to whether we are happy in the relationship and want to continue in it. People change. Relationships change.

Luckily, we always have choice.

Pursuit Not Received

On the flip side, I've worked with couples where it was the women who were not open to being pursued. Some women almost enjoyed rebuffing their partner's advances. It gave them a sense of power and an opportunity for passive-aggressive digs at them. Sometimes, the women had been sexually abused as children and had a deep distrust of men's intentions. Even though they desired the connection and trust of their partner, they couldn't relax and enjoy the attention they did get.

There was one couple where the woman continually rejected her husband no matter what he did. For her, as a young child, her father had left her mother for another woman. Then, for the next fifteen years, all she heard about was how horrible men were from her mother. This dynamic was then brought into her marriage, and she subconsciously viewed her husband in the same light as her father. She could never just relax and receive. Over time, her husband's desire to pursue slowly disappeared, and before long, any honeymoon magic was lost.

If we are the one in the masculine and our partner does not want to be pursued, then this must become an important topic of discussion in the relationship. Are they upset about something? Is it within their relationship? Is it something else? Do they even want this kind of romantic attention or a passionate relationship?

For centuries, we swept these kinds of uncomfortable conversations under the rug and hope that the issue magically disappears. Often, we didn't have the words to explain how we felt if the issue was sexual or post-partum depression or simply a difficult conversation. This was especially necessary where divorce wasn't allowed or disapproved of.

However, today, we can learn how to communicate in kindness. We can go to counselling for help with issues that we can't get to the bottom of by ourselves. We can ask for help. We have many options today.

Till Death Do Us Part

Ironically, the wedding vow "I promise to be with you until death do we part" can often signal the end of all romance. Once we promise that we are never going to leave, something can easily relax inside of each of us. We think, "Well, I can do anything (or nothing) because they aren't going to leave anyway." There is a kind of complacency we can easily fall into once we have that committed relationship. After all, they won't leave because we love each other. Right?

Imagine instead, that our wedding vows included a promise to keep the fires of passion burning—that we would always communicate in kindness and keep the excitement alive for the entirety of our relationship. If we wrote our vows similar to this, we would become very conscious as to whether this was something we actually wanted to get into or not. We might even change "until death do us part" to "until our passion subsides and our paths diverge." Just imagine.

Reverse Polarity in Pursuit

It is interesting to note that if the feminine partner pursues the masculine partner, it seldom works. The masculine often energetically runs away. I don't know why, but this is a dynamic that seldom swaps polarity. On occasion, the feminine pursuing the masculine might be the perfect answer. But most of the time, if the feminine has to pursue, this is where a lot of bitterness and resentment starts to enter a relationship.

If a relationship becomes stagnant, the feminine partner will often start to initiate. They will try to be intimate or plan date nights. But their partner will often push them away and say no.

Of course, as in all pursuit, nobody has to agree to something they don't desire. So, just because the feminine partner wants something, the masculine partner doesn't have to want it as well. However, if the masculine never pursues and leaves it to the feminine to initiate, hard feelings will start to surface in direct and passive-aggressive ways.

The feminine simply wants connection. If they are going to be with each other exclusively, then romantic connection is part of that. If the masculine doesn't pursue, and the feminine pursuing doesn't work either, then the passion in the relationship is sunk.

The next step is dependent on the desire of the feminine partner. If they are content to have a comfortable companionship, then they will just accept that the passionate part of their relationship is over, and they will settle into something more neutral. However, if they desire a dynamic, romantic relationship, then they will have to make another choice.

Dating Dynamics

The dance of pursuit is especially relevant when we are dating and seeking a partner. As we have seen, it is important that it continues in relationships as well. But in dating, this dynamic is more like a mating ritual in the animal kingdom than the effort of keeping the fires alive in a relationship.

Initially, pursuit in dating is the phase where we wonder if they want to be with us. Will there be a relationship at all? For the masculine, there is considerably more risk as to whether the other person will return their desire. For the feminine, there is the fear and frustration of not being pursued or being pursued by someone they aren't attracted to. There are many opportunities for hurt feelings and frustrations here, so it is good to look at it on its own.

THE RISK OF PURSUIT

I once had a boyfriend who was very shy and introverted. We had quite a rocky start because after we met and had a lovely date, he didn't text or try to see me for a while.

Since I love being in the feminine in romance, I didn't pursue him. I just let him go. I figured that being in the masculine wasn't his nature, and that's great. He would find someone who was a better match on the polarity continuum than me. A few weeks later, he messaged me saying, "I don't understand what's happened. Why aren't we talking anymore?"

I responded, "Well, I'm not going to pursue you. That's not my interest, and if it's not your nature, then we probably are not a good match." He said, "No, I want to go out with you. Okay, let me take you out for dinner."

While out for dinner, he asked me what exactly it meant to be in the masculine. I explained that it was like planning dinners and fun things to do together. It was initiating intimacy and giving in the bedroom. He hadn't heard anything like it before, but he said, "Oh, okay. I'm happy to do all that. I'm happy to be in the masculine." We ended up having a lovely relationship.

A few months later, I asked him, "So what exactly happened there? Why didn't you pursue me?" He replied, "Well, I was afraid you'd say no, and I just couldn't handle being rejected."

This is a real thing. Nobody likes being rejected. There is something very challenging about sticking your neck out and pursuing because there is always this risk of rejection.

The key here is that it comes back to having that inner balance and confidence that knows everything will be okay, no matter what happens. And it's not just in relationships. It could be starting a new business, trying something new, or choosing to travel. There is a confidence that says, "I don't know how this is going to work out, but I'm willing to give it a go. I have faith that I have the resilience to handle whatever happens."

That inner confidence and resilience is key.

When Pursuit is Not Desired

Let's say that you see someone whom you would like to pursue, but there isn't any true magnetism. Maybe they look like something your brain desires. Maybe you are just horny, and they are the kind of person that we learned is attractive, who is "this height" or "this body type". You could simply be attracted to that.

If you approach them, and they aren't feeling the same attraction, then they must say, "No, thank you." The challenge is to not take this personally. We have learned a lot of strange ideas through Hollywood and the media about sexual attraction and relationships, like the idea that only good-looking and successful people get great partners. We are also taught that if we look a certain way, everyone will be attracted to us.

This subconsciously sets us up for disappointment. This makes us think that if someone says no to us, then we must not be good-looking or successful enough. We assume that there's something wrong with us because we have been taught that if we were "good enough," then everyone would like us — like the popular people in Hollywood.

However, this is a just shallow story that sells movies. It is also based on the idea that we are always desperate to find a partner because if we don't, we are only half a person. This creates wonderful drama that is great for story plots as it triggers all kinds of emotional responses in the audience, but it has little to do with real life and true human magnetism.

Instead, let's imagine that we don't believe that we are a partial person if we are alone. Let's imagine that we are whole — fully masculine and feminine all on our own. Then, if we approach someone, and they say no, we assume that we read the situation wrong and keep on walking. We don't have to think, "Oh, I'm a loser," or "Of course, they don't like me," or anything like that. It's important that we try. Sometimes it lines up, and sometimes it doesn't. We have to be able to honour the truth of whatever magnetic attraction is there or not.

Sometimes, we mistake a fetish for magnetic attraction. In Naomi Wolf's book *The Beauty Myth,* she addresses our obsession with the beauty of another.

> *"When men are more aroused by symbols of sexuality than by the sexuality of women themselves, they are fetishists. Fetishism treats a part as if it were the whole; men who choose a lover based on her "beauty" alone are treating the woman as a fetish – that is, treating a part of her, her visual image, not even her skin, as if it were her sexual self."*

SEXUAL INTIMACY & DIVINE UNION

This applies to all genders and orientations. Are we magnetically attracted to this person as a whole being? Or are we simply attracted to how they look? Are we turned on by the idea of having sex with them? Are we drawn by the idea of having someone that attractive in our lives?

This comes into play when we might be attracted to someone because they are tall or blonde or muscular or well-endowed. Our minds are so attached to these ideals of beauty that we may not even know how to feel true mutual attraction to another person. The visuals and ideals in our brain override our whole system.

I once went to a tantra speed dating event. As I initially scanned the room, there was one man who caught my eye. Ironically, there was also a little voice inside of me that said "no" (which at the time I was happy to override because he was strikingly handsome).

In one of the exercises, we were blindfolded and placed in front of another person sitting a few inches away. We had to notice whether our body naturally pulled away or leaned towards the other person. We were testing our natural magnetism with no visuals.

As I sat blindfolded before the first man, my body leaned way back. My body was literally repulsed by his energy. When we took off our blindfolds, it was the same man who had caught my eye. My heart knew the truth on sight, but my brain tried to tell me otherwise.

Imagine how different the pursuit game would be if we were able to actually feel whether there was magnetism or not between us and not just follow what our brains wanted.

BAIT & SWITCH

Sometimes, the feminine person will do a bait and switch. They will text, call, pursue, and even make plans with the person they want to date. They will try to make it easy for them because they are attracted to them. There is nothing wrong with this at all, and sometimes it works out brilliantly.

The problem comes if their real hope is that once the other agrees to the date, and they get to know each other, they will be able to back off on all the initiating, and the other person will step into the masculine. However, this seldom works because it isn't how they set it up. They showed the other person right from the beginning that they would pursue them — that they would take the masculine role. And that is exactly what happens. They pursue them, and the other person stays in the feminine.

Of course, we can pursue anyone we want. The question is, what dynamic do you want in the potential relationship? If you want to be in the feminine, but you have to do the pursuing to get them in the relationship to begin with, there's a high chance that you will never be pursued by them at all. They showed their nature right away. They are never going to enjoy making dinner plans or initiating anything in the relationship. Maybe it isn't what they want or it just isn't who they are right now.

Again, we get to do whatever we want. We just have to have full consciousness of what it is we desire in the relationship if we actually get it.

WHAT IF THEY DON'T PURSUE ME?

What do you do if you are interested in someone, but they don't make a move? Well, you can go after them. Lots of people who actually prefer the feminine polarity might say, "I'm not going to sit around and wait for them," which is cool as long as you're happy with being in the masculine role in the relationship. If that is what you want, awesome. If that is not what you want, we have to learn how to be feminine and enjoy being whole and happy.

It comes back to being complete people — with or without a relationship. This is why we aren't just sitting around desperately waiting. This is the difference. If we need a partner to fulfill us, to make us feel beautiful, loved, important, or cherished, then if someone doesn't pay attention to us, we essentially hold our breath until they notice us because, without them, we don't count.

The point of this whole book is to have this masculine-feminine balance within us so that we can be happy. If someone walks by, and they pay attention to us, then maybe we find that there's a natural magnetism between us. That's the thing—we are looking for truth. We're not looking for something that we made up in our minds. We are looking for what is real. Now, if someone walks by, your two poles line up, and something wakes up in both of you, this is a true attraction. If they walk by, and there is no attraction, you realize that they didn't notice and life goes on.

Either there was no magnetism, or even if there was, maybe they were not in a place to act on it. Perhaps they are in a committed relationship. Maybe they have ideas in their head of the person they want, and they are not even noticing real magnetism. One way or the other, they are not available. If their pole doesn't line up with your pole, it isn't there, and this is important for you to honour.

Sometimes we easily get stuck in that maiden archetype who just wants everybody to love her and for everybody to think she is pretty. This is where we have to take a deep breath, step back into our wisdom, and say, "Well, they seem like a nice person. I guess now's not the time for that," and we get on with our life. It is that simple.

Your Personal Journey:

IF YOU'RE IN A RELATIONSHIP NOW:

1. Does the masculine partner pursue the feminine? What does that look like?
2. Does the feminine partner enjoy the advances of the masculine? If yes, awesome. If not, how come? Do they not like what's being offered? Is it a struggle to be in the feminine due to past pain or trauma? What could she do to heal and embrace her feminine?
3. Are the roles often reversed? Does the partner who prefers the feminine have to pursue? Does this work for you both?

4. What would be the ideal pursuit dance in your relationship? What would really stoke the fires of passion for you?

IF YOU'RE DATING AND SEEKING A ROMANCE:

1. If you prefer the masculine polarity, are you comfortable pursuing? Are you okay with people saying no?
2. If you prefer the feminine, are you comfortable being pursued? Are you honest with your yeses and noes?
3. How do you find this masculine and feminine dance playing out in your dating experience? Is it healthy and fun?
4. Are you clear about what kind of relationship you are seeking?

Chapter 15

Leading & Following In Intimacy

He was deep inside of me and gently moving. As I breathed slowly, my inner voice kept saying, "Totally relax." So, I would relax my vagina more. "Relax even more." So, I started relaxing the muscles all around my pelvis. This journey of "Relax even more" continued until I was like a limp doll — like there wasn't a single muscle activated in my whole body.

Then, crazy things started happening inside of me. My whole body was vibrating, although I wasn't moving. I was like a musical instrument, and the sound was coming from between the strings. The more I relaxed, the stronger the vibrations became.

My partner felt all of these vibrations, but it didn't bother his ability to stay with me. Often, when I became orgasmic, it would trigger him to ejaculate. But not this time. The more I vibrated, the more we breathed together. The more I felt his strength, the more I relaxed, and the greater the vibrations.

I have no idea how long we played in these vibrations or where the sensations were coming from, but it felt absolutely other-worldly.

In leading and following, the feminine surrenders to the masculine's lead. The trick is that the masculine surrenders to the union first. This is as important in the bedroom as it is in the example of our cousin the salsa dancer.

SEXUAL INTIMACY & DIVINE UNION

If we want our feminine partner to let down her guard and be able to be completely open and receptive, she must be able to trust that he is paying complete attention to her and not simply satisfying his own needs. If she feels like he is just serving his own needs, it is actually not wise for her to let her guard down. She doesn't know where he is coming from. And because he is actually feeding his own needs, she as a whole person is irrelevant. She is simply the object of his fantasy, pleasure, and desire.

The first time a man completely surrendered himself to me, I couldn't believe the effect on my body. As he approached me, he bowed his head, saying, "I am so honoured to be with you." As he touched my arms, I instantly opened to him—mind, body and spirit. All my skin came alive. As he felt my energy go completely soft, he then stepped into the masculine lead, picked me up, carried me to the bedroom, and the magnetic pull between us was absolutely insane.

This pattern has continued. The strongest men and the greatest lovers have always intuitively surrendered themselves to the experience first. After that, everything just flows magically.

Inspiration & Manifestation

This is an important dynamic for both leaders and followers in lovemaking because we don't want to bring our brains into the bedroom. Some say that the brain is an important sexual organ. This can definitely be true in the pursuit and arousal phase. However, our brains also hold all of our fears, walls, techniques, and expectations—all of which stand in the way of union. Our brains are actually the primary barrier to true connection and merging. It is our bodies and souls that we need to connect. To do this, we must lead through inspiration and intuition.

To begin, we want to fully drop in with our partner. We want to feel them. We want to breathe with them. We want to feel their presence. Then, with a quiet mind, we wait for a desire or idea to rise (feminine inspiration) within us. We then manifest (masculine) what comes to us. It could be a touch, a position, or a kiss.

Inspiration might appear as a vision in our mind of a position or a caress. It could be a feeling or a hunch that keeps repeating inside of us. The key is to be open to whatever comes because it might not be what you expect. Our brains work on patterns of what we have experienced before and what we think we know about ourselves and our partner. However, intuition is working with the current moment. It is considering the whole. It is considering things that you may not even consciously know about. This is what makes it such an adventure—to almost walk blindly in total faith that your intuition will guide you somewhere you've never been before.

Although it is the masculine partner who is leading, initially, both partners will be listening within. Every lovemaking session is a journey of connection. So, as both partners transition from their separate states to being connected to each other, either partner may feel inspired to move into a particular position or touch the other in a certain way. As their connection solidifies, their polarity will increase, and they will start to flow naturally together. The acting upon their inspiration won't be so obvious. The energy of lovemaking will just flow.

There will be times that you shift in and out of union. This is natural. Energy flows like a sine wave—rising and falling. The key is to just listen within, do what you feel, and enjoy whatever experience comes.

The Joy of Leading in Intimacy

I once met a man on a retreat who was a BDSM Dom who was really lovely, and we ended up chatting all night in the hot tub. He was asking me about the masculine and feminine in tantra. He was accustomed to a masculine-feminine dynamic, where his feminine partner may be tied up while he was being dominant. He wanted to know the difference between what he experienced in his world and what one might experience in tantra.

I asked him to gently move my arm. We were in a hot tub so it was easy to relax my body in the water and have him move me. As he moved me, my challenge was to fully let him, to let down my guards, release all control, and trust him to move me gently. If he moved me too quickly, I would tense up. If he slowed down and paid full attention to me, I could relax into him. The more I could trust him to stay focused, the more connected we became. The more connected we became, the more I could relax into anything he did with my body.

Soon, we were just floating in a beautiful cloud of energy. He was still moving me, but that wasn't how it felt. It was like we were both just flowing together—giver and receiver had disappeared. We just floated and flowed blissfully for the next couple of hours.

We realized that there can be a thrill in being tied up and controlled. It combines many other emotional responses that can be very exciting. If it is done in kindness, there is definitely connection and trust. However, you are always inherently separate. There is no question as to who is the dominant and who is the submissive.

What we experienced in that hot tub was union. With each movement, breath, and moment of responsibility or surrender, our energies merged together. In the end, there was no sense of separation at all. The polarities had collapsed into One. We had total union.

Leading in the Bedroom

Leading is not just deciding what will happen next. It is also about reading our partner. It is about sensing what is going on, making the moves, and initiating the energy that will flow through both of you. It is a wonderful combination of what your partner loves and what you love. Both of you are whole beings. Neither is subservient to the other. We are simply taking different roles with the intention of pleasurable connection and union.

What can be challenging for the masculine partner is that their feminine partner is always changing. If the feminine is a woman, she is chemically different every day of the month. Her sexual organs change position with her hormone levels. Regardless of gender, the feminine partner flows in all the feminine qualities—

chaos, surrender, wildness, vulnerability, and deep truth. This means that they will always be a little bit different than they were last time. They will have had realizations and aha moments. They will feel differently inside than yesterday. They will be in a whole new place.

Of course, the masculine partner is also a different person than yesterday. Everyone is constantly growing and changing, but in the dynamic of leading and following, it is the masculine partner who must initiate a connection with this other human who may be radically different than the last time.

What a wonderful challenge! What a wonderful adventure to get to explore this person you love in a new state, on new terrain. Where are they today? What do I feel from them? How does my new energy blend with their reality?

This is where lovemaking stays alive, dynamic, and potent! The feminine fully drops into their sensitive, open, reality, and the masculine explores every inch of it. It is so exciting!

Following in Lovemaking

Releasing in lovemaking is such a wonderful gift. It has the potential to open parts of us that we have never felt before.

It's like floating on the water. If we are good at floating, we can relax our bodies and just float around effortlessly, but we cannot let go completely. There is always a small part of us paying attention to our surroundings and staying aware that we are floating on water so that we don't fall asleep or let our head go under.

There is a beautiful practice called Watsu where the masculine partner stands in the water with the feminine partner's head on their shoulder. The masculine then supports the feminine's body and gently floats them all around. The dynamic of releasing and fully trusting this person is the first joy. Then to feel the water caressing your body while you lie 100% trusting another person brings your body to a whole new level of bliss.

In lovemaking, we will release to the same degree that our partner is attentively leading. We will always be in balance with each other. As the masculine gains confidence in their lead, and our connection grows deeper, the feminine will relax more and more and more.

Listening Within

Along this feminine journey, there are times when we struggle to follow. Maybe a trust issue from a previous partner comes up, and we start to close down.

This is a beautiful moment to ask for guidance from within. Ask for inspiration. Maybe you need your partner to slow down, speed up, or do something differently. Maybe you need to be held for a while. Maybe you need to talk or cry.

Intimacy is an opportunity for many different kinds of experiences. It isn't just about wild and passionate sex, or tantric intimacy. It is the blending of souls. You truly never know what is going to come up. Although you are in the feminine, and your focus is to enjoy the blissful follow, you are still a human being who is also the wild feminine deeply connected to her chaos. Within that chaos are many mysteries, hidden feelings, and unexpected joys.

So, having guidance along the way is definitely how we navigate this exciting path!

Your Personal Journey:

Strengthening the Feminine

1. How easily do you release in lovemaking? If it's a challenge, why? Are there past experiences that hold you back?
2. Have you experienced a strong and attentive lead before? Have you experienced unhealthy leads?
3. Do you like to lead sometimes? What does that feel like? What do you learn about following by leading once in a while?
4. Do you trust your intuition to guide you in following?

Strengthening the Masculine

1. Is leading easy for you? Do you trust your intuition to guide you?
2. What would give you more confidence in leading in the bedroom? What stops you?
3. Do you enjoy the adventure of discovering your partner anew each time?
4. Does your partner ever like to lead? What do you learn about leading when you get to completely follow?

SEXUAL INTIMACY & DIVINE UNION

CHAPTER 16
GIVING & RECEIVING IN INTIMACY

*"Rivers of power flowing everywhere.
Fields of magnetism relating everything.
This is your origin. This is your lineage.
The current of creation is right here,
Coursing through subtle channels,
Animating this very form.
Follow the gentle touch of life,
Soft as the footprint of an ant,
As tiny sensations open to vastness.
Power sings as it flows,
Electrifies the organs of sensing,
Becomes liquid light,
Nourishes your entire being.
Celebrate the boundary
Where streams join the sea,
Where body meets infinity."*
LORIN ROCHE, The Radiance Sutras

The Joy of Giving Sexually

Imagine your feminine partner is before you. This is the beautiful person that you get to explore. Who are they? How are they feeling? You wonder what your partner would love to do. You listen within. You begin by holding them in your arms, just breathing together.

As you feel them nuzzle into you, you begin stroking their hair. You feel them breathe more deeply, so you continue, following your intuition, and loving every second.

Giving is easy. The key is to release our minds and just let our bodies make love — to allow our bodies to be magnetically drawn to wherever our partner's body calls us.

How do we do this? Releasing any goals we may have, letting go of expectations (of ourselves and our partner), and remembering why we are doing this. There is so much joy and fun and pleasure to be had!

When we come to lovemaking with a light heart, we are naturally relaxed and fully present. This lets us truly feel the skin of our lover. We feel their skin as if we have never touched a human before. When we are thankful for this beautiful person in our lives, we slow down even more, making our touch very magnetic and full of even more pleasure.

There have been a lot of fears placed within us that we will do it wrong or that we may not be a great lover. However, these are all from the world of separation. This is where the goal is to get pleasure for yourself (separate), pleasure your partner (separate), or prove your lovemaking prowess (separate again).

The journey to union is completely different. There is no such thing as a "great lover." There are no "right" or "wrong" things to do. All that matters is that we are responding to this beautiful person beside us in the present moment. With every genuine response, our connection becomes deeper, and we continue to flow in that energy.

Choosing Your Palette

Every time we are intimate with our feminine partner, we learn what they enjoy and what brings them pleasure. What our partner loves is very important.

The things that they love become your palette for lovemaking. Of course, this palette is filled in by trial and error. You try something and notice the response. If it's positive, it's added to the palette. If they don't like it, we try something else.

This is where our partner must give very clear responses. If we think that we have to let them feel like they are "doing it right," even when we are not enjoying it, things will not work in our favour. For the feminine, faking orgasm is as old as time. However, in order to have a true connection, honesty is really important. Sometimes we are in sync, everything flows effortlessly, and it is obvious what would please our partner. However, because our feminine partner is by nature wild and unpredictable, it is sometimes helpful to receive an indication from them as to what would feel wonderful right now.

From this pleasurable and light-hearted dance, our palette continues to fill (a bit more in each lovemaking session until forever). Then, when we are choosing how to give or what the next step is, we check in intuitively and choose from our palette.

Flowing Energy

When our feminine partner truly responds to our touch, energy starts to move. This energy flowing between us is where pure bliss lives. We both have our own unique energetic DNA sequence. As we connect and merge with them, a whole different pattern can be experienced.

The more we touch and feel that connection, the more electricity is there. The role of the giver is to give in this way consistently so that the other feels safe to completely relax and receive. The more they relax and receive, the more energy that comes through our hands, our mouths, and our bodies to give. As they feel this and release, the energy flowing through them will amp up and up and up.

This energy doesn't have to be frenetic. It can be very relaxed. You could be just lying on the bed, your partner slowly caressing you, and you are melting into their touch. Or it could be a much stronger touch or sexual intercourse. It is all about the connection. It is all about reading whatever is desired at that moment.

Giving Completely

Once we have the energy circuit connected, and the energy is all flowing in one direction, the next step is to increase the power. How do we do that? By giving all that we've got and holding nothing back. There's a saying in sports that we want "to leave everything on the field." This is also our goal in lovemaking.

Lovemaking is a natural movement based on our desires to connect with one another. There is no need for thoughts or fears. These will only put up barriers and turn lovemaking into something it is not — something we want to accomplish, get something from, or be satisfied by. This might be sexual intercourse, but it is not lovemaking.

We are made for love. We are made to give it without abandon. Why would we hold anything back? If we have never experienced flowing love before, we may not know what this feels like. So, we just go through the motions because we can't imagine letting our guards down enough with anyone (including ourselves) to love completely.

However, the joy comes in the flow of love. This is palpable. You can feel it. It is like an energy force drawing you together, flowing between you, and guiding your motions all at the same time.

Receiving in Intimacy

When I first became single, dating was quite a challenge. Although I didn't want to be in the masculine, I tended to take over in the bedroom because I didn't want to just have normal sex. I wanted it to be slow, connected, and tantric, and most of the men I had dated had never experienced this. So, I tended to be in the masculine, controlling what was happening, whether I wanted to or not.

Then I met the lovely man who took me out for dinner in Chapter 16. One time, while making love, I started taking over when he stopped me and said, "Katrina, you wanted me to be in the masculine. Let me. Let me give to you. Just relax and receive."

I was so surprised that I still had some resistance to this. However, there was something about his kindness that just stopped me in my tracks. I had to learn how to fully relax and receive. As I looked into his eyes and started tearing up, he said, "There is nothing else I would rather be doing than giving to you right now."

I realized that I had much more to learn about receiving. Maybe it was due to lovers in the past who had actually wanted to receive themselves. They didn't want to just give, or they were only giving in order to receive later. However, this man loved to give, and the more he did it, the more I believed him. It didn't take too long before I could truly relax and trust that he really wanted to be doing this, and I could open myself to fully receive.

There was something about this man that finally let me trust and take my hands off the steering wheel completely. From here, I was able to receive more in all aspects of my life. I trusted that intuition would guide me, that help would appear when I needed it, and that I didn't have to always be the one giving.

I could finally relax and start receiving from the world around me.

When the Masculine Enters

Receiving in intimacy also shows up in intercourse when the masculine enters the feminine (through whatever means). Historically, the timing of entry has been up to the masculine partner. Even today, many feminine partners don't know that it is actually up to the feminine. When they are loved and given to, the feminine body will open naturally.

This works with women and men. In a woman, the vagina opens and becomes magnetically negative, which means it becomes a bit like a vacuum, pulling in toward her. In heterosexual relationships, they will come to a point in the intimacy where she will feel this desire as her vagina becomes a negative, magnetic vacuum. She will want you inside of her NOW.

For males in the feminine polarity, when they feel loved, caressed, and connected to a truly masculine partner, their anus will be able to relax completely. They will open in very similar ways… all at the hands of a loving masculine partner.

THE HONOUR OF BEING RECEIVED COMPLETELY

Sometimes feminine partners struggle with receiving because they feel like they aren't doing anything. They feel like they are just receiving, "just lying there." This is because we don't understand the value of fully receiving another human being.

I remember making love with a man once when I realized that he wasn't giving his whole self to me. He was holding back. I tried to coax him gently to give all of himself, but he couldn't.

As I lay there, I realized that being received sexually is similar to how we are received in the world. Let's say that this man felt comfortable giving 80% of who he was to me in intimacy, but he was going to hold 20% back. Perhaps this is also what he gave to the world. Maybe he feared judgement and didn't let most people see all of who he was. Maybe there was an inherent distrust in others that made him want to "keep his cards close."

I wondered if some people were only able to give 20% of themselves in the world. Did this translate to how they made love as well?

However, I also had to look at myself. Was I 100% open to receiving him? In life and in the bedroom? Were there parts of him that I judged and didn't like? Maybe I was the one holding back. Maybe I was only allowing 80% of him inside of me. Maybe it had nothing to do with him.

So, I imagined what it would feel like to fully receive this man — in life, energetically, and in intimacy. As I leaned into this, I felt myself open even more. I felt more guards fall away and allow more of him in — in and out of the bedroom. Slowly, he was able to give more and I was able to receive more. This opened us up to experiencing new levels in our lovemaking. We were able to open doors that were previously closed. We were able to feel more subtle connections between us. We got to experience complete union.

I realized what an important role the receiver could be in someone's life. Imagine the masculine partner knowing that this person receives them completely — every ounce of them. Not only do they receive and accept them, but they love them.

Just imagine how healing and powerful that is!

Divine Union

It is when the masculine and feminine come together that all creation happens. Giving and receiving in intimacy is one of the most beautiful dynamics to explore this idea.

Let's imagine that the masculine partner is Divine Energy, and the feminine partner is the Divine Container. The key to creation is to fill the container with the energy of the Universe.

When you give to someone in love and kindness, you can feel their energy expand. As you caress their body, they will relax, and you can feel them start to change. It's like their body starts to light up and fill the room. Their container expands. As they expand, it is like a vacuum is created, drawing the masculine in even more.

As you continue to give, and they receive you more and more, the energy of the feminine becomes bigger and bigger. If you gaze upon them at this point, you will notice that they don't look like themselves. They may look younger or completely different and cosmic. When they look at you, they will find the same thing. You both will have been transformed.

At this point, you are simply the Divine Masculine and the Divine Feminine. You are no longer your personalities. One is pure masculine/giving energy and the other is pure feminine/receptive energy. There are no more preferences in how one likes to give or receive. You are both just pure energy of the Universe.

Perhaps we are playing in different dimensions or different energy states. As much as we may be touching, caressing, kissing, or in intercourse, it all becomes quite secondary to the energetic experience of this divine creation of a brand new energy.

Your Personal Journey:

Strengthening the Feminine

1. Are you able to fully receive in intimacy (regardless of polarity preference)?
2. Can you relax completely to allow your container to expand?
3. Have you ever been able to trust someone to give you what you desire in intimacy?
4. Are you honest in your feedback as to what you like and don't like?

Strengthening the Masculine

1. Do you enjoy giving to a lover? If not, what do you think gets in your way?
2. Are you able to "leave it all on the field" or do you tend to hold back?
3. Do you enjoy turning off your mind and just letting your body make love with your partner?
4. Can you imagine being received 100% by someone else? How would that feel?

Chapter 17
Structure & Chaos in Intimacy

We are making love, and my only desire is to relax completely. I want to surrender every cell of my body to him. As I surrender, he is moving in and out of me. My orgasmic state begins. I start to feel the wildness. The chaos starts to overwhelm me.

Suddenly, I have a vision of being a siren in the water taunting him to come into the water with me. I want to make him explode, to lose control, to cum. But I don't really want him to. I want him to fight me. I want to feel his strength. I want the tug-of-war. I want the chance to be even wilder.

I say to him, "Imagine I'm in the water. There is a rope. You must hold onto the rope to keep me safe." Then I tell him about my siren's desire to pull him in. To overwhelm him.

He says that he won't be pulled in. He becomes stronger. He will take over. He passionately kisses me. He owns me with his vajra (penis). I am the one being overwhelmed. The more he kisses me, the wilder I get. The wilder I get, the more presence his vajra has as it goes deeper.

We find our rhythm. He has to get bigger. He has to stay in his masculine. He can't get lost in my chaos. He has to keep driving the boat. He has to listen within for guidance and strength. I will pull him in if he doesn't.

I got the tug-of-war I wanted. It became wild and furious. We pulled hard in opposite directions, fully trusting the other to stay connected until the final crescendo peaked, and we fell into a sweaty pile of bodies, heavy breathing, and total bliss.

In this dynamic, each person is holding an entirely different kind of energy. The energies are playing off of each other to create a bigger and bigger experience.

Let's say the masculine starts to arouse the feminine. The feminine begins to move from her centred whole place into that feminine, sensual, and wild place. Her body begins to awaken with sensual desire. The masculine continues to caress her, opening her up, allowing her to release the masculine stronghold that she normally needs in order to get along in the outside world.

As she drops her masculine structure and order, his structure becomes stronger. He digs within to find a deeper strength. As he becomes stronger, she knows it is safe to become wilder. The wilder she becomes, the deeper and stronger he becomes.

The amazing thing about this is that it doesn't even matter if you polarize to 100%. The whole dance is exciting and wild for both people at any degree of polarization. However, if you do continue to polarize, moving toward the limit, one becoming wilder and wilder and the other stronger and stronger, you both start to lose touch with reality. The spinning top starts to spin at an incredible pitch.

As we initially explore this, we will often slow down to catch our bearings. We are not accustomed to feeling so out of control (and if there is a male involved, there is the fear of ejaculating), so we slow the spinning top down a little bit while we gather ourselves. The more we play with this polarity, the further out we go. And once we can go all the way, we lose ourselves completely in the experience. It is like we are holding onto each other's bodies for dear life and flying through the unknown together.

This is where our physical bodies disappear completely, and we experience something beyond description.

Diving into the Feminine

Let's talk about chaos, wildness, and the unknown in sexual intimacy.

This is where we get to feel so alive. We get to play in the part of us that loves the unknown, wants to explore something new, and wants to live at a very deep and primal level. We seldom get to experience this in our tamed lives where there are many rules out there that we have to live within.

Even if we are wild in our day-to-day life, there are always some restrictions of some kind. Even being in a physical body is a restriction. However, in intimacy, we can be wide open to chaos and the unknown. We are in an infinite playing field where anything is possible.

PLAYING IN THE UNKNOWN

Chaos in intimacy, on a practical level, is not knowing what is going to happen next.

It is easy to take what has happened in the past and try to repeat it. This could be with the same partner, or if we are with a new partner, we will naturally try what has worked previously. We assume that if it worked before, it will likely work again. Unfortunately, as pleasurable as it may be, we will not expand into what else is possible because we are just going through an old pattern in our brain.

Instead, imagine that you've never been with this person. Maybe you've never been with anyone. This opens up brand-new possibilities. It creates a blank slate. Anything could happen. This is true chaos. This is trusting that there is more out there than what we have experienced in the past. All we have to do is be 100% present so that we can hear guidance for what to do next.

When we listen within, ideas might arise that maybe we weren't expecting—a desire to do something or say something that makes you think, "Oh, I can't say that.", "I've never done that!", or "What would others think?" You play with it in your mind a bit, and then you think, "Okay, I'm going to try." You do it, and the whole experience flies somewhere wonderful you've never been before.

Chaos is what we get to explore in intimacy. By listening to our intuition and instinct, we have added the element of wildness. It means that we don't have to look a certain way. We don't have to make or not make certain sounds. We don't have to act a certain way. We can do and be anything. We can scream, moan, and writhe if we want. And if we don't like what's happening, we can change it. We can change positions. We can move. We can do something else. We must always be open to whatever our body wants.

We can express the sounds that our body wants to make. Not sounds from our head or thoughts, but the actual primal 'ah' sounds that our bodies are making. This adds this whole element to our sensual flow. We don't know what is going to come out of our mouth. We don't know what our body's going to do. This is where we are exploring something new.

It is an infinite world. Anything is possible. And as soon as we step outside the known and the things we have done, we start carving new paths of possibility. This is how sexual intimacy, even with the same partner, never gets old. If we are paying attention and allowing for the wildness, everything is always new. Every time is like the first time.

It's important to note that wildness doesn't mean craziness and out-of-control passion all of the time either. It simply means there are no rules. It could mean spooning and being completely silent. There is great magic that can happen in stillness. You can't plan it. It just all of a sudden happens. You might be doing this crazy thing, and then all of a sudden, you stop. There is an energy between you that is palpable, and you swim in this incredible magnetism. This is also wildness.

This is why we can't give an equation for experiencing a tantric orgasmic state. It is only through the wild that we find it. All of a sudden, you will do something and have an experience that you've never had before. You may never be able to replicate it. You just have to trust the wildness to take you wherever it wants to go.

Power of Masculine Stillness in Intimacy

I remember this one lovely man who would often ejaculate if I got really chaotic, wild, and orgasmic. So, if I felt him getting too close to his edge, I would pull my orgasm back. He could always tell when I started to hold back, and he'd say, "I don't want you to pull back like that. I want you to fully experience it. What can I do to not cum?" I told him that he could practise contracting his PC muscle, but really, he just had to find the switch inside of him. He needed to turn off the primal need to ejaculate where has have no power or control and turn on the switch that gives him all of the power.

A few days later, he came back, and again, we were making love. I could feel myself heading into that wild, unbridled, orgasmic state. I was afraid that he was going to cum, so I started pulling back. He said, "What are you doing?" I replied, "I'm pulling back. I don't want you to cum." He responded, "I've got you. Go. Go right to the end of yourself. Don't worry about me."

What? I almost married him right on the spot. I was able to fly, to explore, to lose myself without any worry about him at all.

This is the beautiful marriage of structure and chaos. To be able to hold space for someone to just go wild and lose themselves is incredible. We are often so structured in our lives, having to look the right way, say the right things, and be responsible, that to get to fly right to the end of yourself and beyond changes you from the inside out.

What's even more exciting is that this is a shared experience when we are in union. My partner also got to experience this unbridled passion because we were energetically connected. Just like electricity, the power runs through the whole circuit. Everything I was experiencing — that wildness, that absolutely ecstatic, chaotic orgasm — we both experienced through his inner stronghold and stillness within.

ORGASM VS EJACULATION

It is important to note that orgasm and ejaculation are not the same things. They often occur at the same time because we only understand a procreative style of sex. In all genders and orientations, we normally to aim for a kind of ejaculation created by friction. With stimulation, you build and build and build, and then you orgasm and ejaculate at the same time. However, they are actually separate things.

If you find the stronghold within you to control the physical ejaculation, you have the opportunity to experience orgasm through your whole body instead of just the genitals. Ejaculation is perfect for procreation. It is perfect when you want to inseminate an egg. However, beyond any kind of procreative desire, we can use this energy, move it through us, and have this ejaculatory orgasmic experience together. In Taoist traditions, unless you desire children, ejaculation is considered a waste of energy. Why not move that energy between you and energize each other? This nourishes both people energetically and physically.

Of course, there are no rules. Simultaneous ejaculation and orgasm are also very pleasurable and wonderful. It's just nice to know that there are many options out there.

Your Personal Journey:

STRENGTHENING THE FEMININE

1. Can you imagine allowing yourself to go totally wild? In lovemaking? Anywhere else in life?
2. Are you comfortable allowing sounds to rise out of your body during lovemaking?
3. How comfortable are you with the unknown? In life? In intimacy?

4. Does the idea of going right to the end of yourself excite you?

STRENGTHENING THE MASCULINE

1. Do you have a strong stillness within you?
2. Can you imagine holding your partner energetically in their wildness? What would that look like for you? (I'm conscious that the example I gave was heterosexual. Perhaps there are many other ways to hold our partner's chaos in other couplings.)
3. Do you enjoy the adventure of becoming stronger inside to witness and eventually experience your partner's orgasmic chaos?

SEXUAL INTIMACY & DIVINE UNION

SECTION V

A Deeper Dive Into the Masculine & Feminine

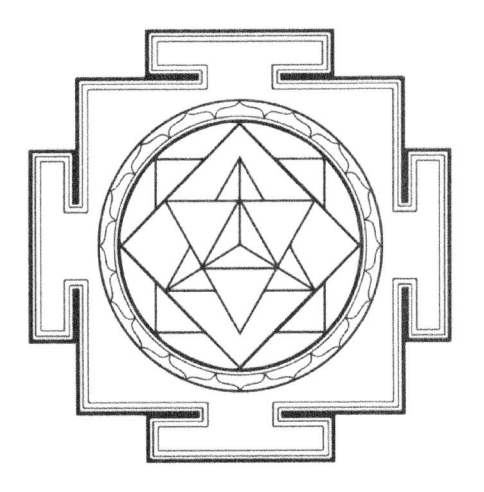

CHAPTER 18

Archetypes of the Masculine & Feminine

*"Understanding of life begins with
the understanding of patterns."*
FRITJOF CAPRA

Sometimes, archetypes are described as being either masculine or feminine. We imagine that a king archetype is masculine, and a queen is feminine. This is because we have interpreted these archetypes in the context of our world of separation and domination. However, if we are to understand these as divine archetypes, then we must consider them as perfectly balanced masculine-feminine and who shift to whatever polarity is necessary depending on the situation.

These archetypes are very helpful when looking at our masculine and feminine dynamics because we can see the separation, the domination, the limitations, and where these patterns appear in our lives and romantic relationships.

King/Queen Archetype

For the sake of simplicity, I am going to use the example of the king here. You could easily replace king with queen depending on the person's gender.

Let's look at two kinds of kings—the Tyrant King and the Benevolent King.

A DEEPER DIVE INTO THE MASCULINE & FEMININE

The tyrant king lives in separation from his people and in separation from his own inner feminine. He desires the power of the position. All must serve him. The people's taxes go to him. Their adoration must be focused on him. He is not concerned with the needs of his kingdom. His kingdom is simply there to serve him.

This is not a masculine archetype. This is the archetype of the broken soul who craves power to fill a void within. This shows the complete lack of connection to their inner feminine, their hurt inner child, the emotions they never listened to, and the person who feels alone and separate from the world.

We easily see this dynamic play out in governments, schools, churches, relationships, and families where whoever is "in charge" is there to be served by the others. The masculine-feminine dynamic is flipped because those in the feminine must serve the masculine. The feminine partner is there to serve the masculine partner. The children must act properly. The parishioners must pay their dues. The people must pay their taxes.

Now let's look at the Benevolent King. His role is to serve his kingdom. He maintains armies to protect his people from marauders. He ensures that there is food for everyone. He listens deeply to the needs of those in his care so that he may provide a great life for them. He takes care of all of his people.

Because he is connected to his own inner feminine, he intrinsically understands the needs of his people. His masculine happily serves his feminine, and that same joy and balance exist in his kingdom as well.

Being in the arms of a benevolent king or queen makes us feel loved, cherished, and safe. With every step, the masculine and the feminine partners become stronger, happier, and more expansive.

Prostitute-Slave Archetype

This archetype often goes with the tyrant king archetype.

This is the flipped feminine archetype where we believe that it is our role to give and ask for nothing in return. We must serve and do whatever the other desires. We have no power, no autonomy, and no sense of self because our entire being is focused on serving our "king". We believe that others have the right to ask for whatever they want, and we must give it to them. We must consider their opinion above our own thoughts and emotions.

This can appear in many places. It can be in students serving their teachers or guru but having no power themselves. It can be in relationships, where one person is in the prostitute/slave archetype, and the other is the king/queen. They are thrown into the old-fashioned powerlessness of the feminine, while actually serving the masculine.

It is a common dynamic in pornography where the women serve the men. This can create challenges for people watching a lot of porn and then desiring connection and wonderful intimacy. Because the dynamics are flipped, true connection, love, and ecstasy are not possible. Each person is just an object. No true energy is flowing.

We can end up in the prostitute archetype because our partner pays the bills, and we feel that we owe them something for this. Maybe we are raised in a culture where you have to have sex with someone because you are married, whether you want to or not. Maybe you must go to work each day and put up with bad treatment without defending yourself or quitting because that is just what you have to do.

This is not an example of being feminine. It isn't even unhealthy or broken feminine. It is a complete lack of the masculine. As the masculine shrinks, so does the feminine. So, we simply become very small. It soon becomes enslavement, and we are powerless.

This is the counterpart to the tyrant king or queen because tyrants need slaves in order to exist. Neither are masculine nor feminine. This is just a have-and-have-not scenario. It serves no one—neither party is grown, fulfilled, healed, or complete in this relationship.

The Father/Daughter Archetype

Here, the masculine partner enjoys being the caregiver and their feminine partner is more like a child. "Here's your money. I've planned all this for you. I've organized this for you. You don't have to worry about anything." They are the saviour. They are the knight on the white horse. They fix everything. They provide everything, and they take great joy in it.

This matches their feminine partner because she wants to be cared for. Maybe they are seeking a father figure. Maybe they feel they can't make decisions on their own. Or maybe they don't want the responsibility of leaving the childhood stage, and this is a way to not have to progress into adulthood.

For others who don't want to be treated as a child, this becomes a great challenge when they find themselves with someone who wants to place them in that child role. It could just be a default role to which the masculine partner is accustomed, and all you need is a conversation to clear it up. However, it is also possible that, unconsciously, they desire the power that this father-role brings. They do not like being questioned. They like holding the purse strings. They like knowing that you are dependent on them. It creates a kind of job security.

On the flip side, a feminine may try to fit a new partner into the father role. They may want them to provide for them financially. They might feign weakness to make their partner step up and take care of them.

In both of these scenarios, the people are not growing into their wholeness. They are playing out familiar power dynamics to feel safe and secure. They are diving into one side of the polarity and staying there.

Something has stopped both of their growth patterns. An actual child is in the feminine because they are not fully formed yet. They need protection to safely grow into an adult. An adult only cares for them because they genuinely need it. These are true masculine and feminine dynamics.

All else is a kind of charade where one pretends to be needy, and the other pretends to save and protect them. Although it may truly meet both partners' need for co-dependency and provide a kind of safety, no kind of intimate union is possible here.

Mother/Son Dynamic

You often will see this in heterosexual couples, but the same energetic pattern appears in same-sex couples, as well.

I have worked with many women who have been married a long time and say, "Well, I have four children if you include the one I married." This is a classic mother-son dynamic. Many women, after they get divorced, decide not to get into new relationships because "they don't want to have to take care of another man." It's like this dynamic is so ingrained they don't believe that anything else is possible.

These women often find men who happily fall into the son role. They scold their partner when they do something wrong. Their "masculine" partner rebels against her. The "feminine" will cook and clean and do their laundry and then be angry because he didn't clean up after himself. The masculine partner may then sulk and go to their room, waiting for the mother-figure's maternal instincts to kick in and either get angrier or forget the whole thing even happened.

Note: I am referring to the woman as the feminine and the man as the masculine because these are the roles that they, in their hearts, would like to be in... even though they are playing out the opposites.

The challenge is that the masculine partner is unconsciously seeking nurturing even though they might be acting like an angry teenager, and the feminine partner doesn't know how else to act in a relationship except to be the scolding and controlling mother.

As a side note, when I was first married in 1993, I remember older women telling me, "Well, a mother raises a boy so far. Then it is the wife's job to raise him the rest of the way." I took this to heart. I didn't know any better. I had always heard that boys mature more slowly than girls. Maybe it was acceptable for men to act any way they wanted whereas women had to grow up more quickly.

In my marriage, this meant that I took care of his feelings and I didn't rock the boat by sharing mine. I didn't think he could handle it. I was always trying to find the high road and never expecting him to. In hindsight, I realize how insulting this was to him. He was a hard-working, full-grown man who didn't ask to be treated like a child. I could easily have acted differently, and we both would have had the chance for a very different relationship.

We can see how challenging it is if someone desires this archetypal dynamic. The masculine wants their partner to take care of them like a mother would—wanting them to cook the meals, clean the house, do the laundry, and spare their feelings when they're upset. Maybe it is all they've ever seen, or maybe it's laziness and the lack of desire to grow up.

On the flip side, a feminine may want to coddle and take care of their partner. This can easily come from centuries of this being the only "real value" of a woman. A woman was judged based on her ability to care for her family and husband. Many women will easily fall into this role by default, believing it is their duty and that they can't do anything else. In order to break out of this generational pattern, the feminine partner will have to find a new journey in life that isn't centred on caring for a partner.

Your Personal Journey:

1. Have you ever fallen into the king archetype? Do you know anyone who enjoys being a tyrant king or a benevolent queen?
2. Can you relate to the prostitute/slave archetype? Are there certain relationships where this seems to come out?
3. Have you ever seen the father/daughter archetype played out? In your own life or others?
4. Have you experienced or seen the mother/son dynamic?

Chapter 19

Strengthening Our Masculine

*"Masculinity is not something given to you,
but something you gain.
And you gain it by winning small battles with honor."*
NORMAN MAILER

This applies to all genders and all polarity preferences. This is about our ability to be masculine out in the world, with other people, in intimate relationships, and within ourselves.

It is important to remember that we always want to be in balance. If our masculine is weak, then our feminine will be equally weak. On our journey to strengthen our masculine, there may be times when we need to nurture our feminine. We need to honour our intuition. We need to heal what has been broken. We need to allow space for chaos. We need to allow for flow within. All these things must be nurtured.

For example, it is hard to give as a masculine if we are empty. If we had a difficult childhood and didn't receive the love, support, and security that a child needs, we may continue to need this as an adult. However, this is something that we must satisfy ourselves. We must find a way to heal this without falling into one of the archetypes mentioned above. We must fill our cup before we can give to others.

If we prefer to be in the masculine role in a relationship, then we have to be connected to our own feminine if we want to fully connect with a partner. Otherwise, we will not understand and be intimidated by their feminine. All the reasons that you aren't connecting with your own feminine will come between you and your romantic partners until you connect within yourself.

So, the feminine is important for sure, but this chapter is about strengthening our masculine. And the only way to do that is through doing.

Strengthening Through Doing

How do we strengthen the masculine? The answer is always doing. The masculine is energy — the energy of action. There is no talking about it. There is no philosophizing about it. It must be done. It is the energy that rises inside of us in the act of doing that increases our masculine.

It could be asking people, "What can I do to help? What can I do to make this happen? How can I support this?" And then do it. It is not about talking. It is not about making to-do lists. It is the action of doing. It is going out into the community and helping.

If we have felt emasculated in our lives, then any masculine act of helping, giving, holding space, or protection strengthens the confidence within us. It makes us know that we can do what we desire. It really is within us.

It is about following through. It is about making plans with people and showing up 100% of the time. It is about volunteering — anything that fills a need in the community. Or if someone is hurting, then you hold space for them. You say, "I'm here for you. I've got you."

It is only through doing.

This applies to ourselves as well. If our inner masculine has struggled, then maybe our protector has to rise and say "no" more often. Maybe we need to step up and say, "You know what? I am going to do yoga every day. I'm going to get past this weird block that is stopping me."

The Chinese proverb "Talk doesn't cook rice" could be the mantra for anyone who wants to strengthen their masculine. It is only the action of doing that changes the visceral memory in our body that makes us know that we will always show up for ourselves.

In relationships, when we get accustomed to always showing up no matter what, we walk with the confidence that we know we are always going to hold up our end of the bargain. We are always going to be our part of the whole. There is great confidence and joy in that.

Trusting Our Inner Masculine

Sometimes, we have a lot of difficulty trusting our own masculine. For example, in the dynamic of inspiration and manifestation, we might decide that we want to get up each day and go running. Our masculine side steps up and makes a plan to do it. We wake up in the first morning to get started, and instead of heading out the door, we say "Nah, I don't want to run this morning."

What happened? Our feminine had a desire to be more active and our masculine rose up and made the plan. Why didn't we do it?

It could be that our masculine is used to just talking and not doing. It's easy to make a plan on paper. It just requires a bit of mental effort. The challenge is to do it in reality. In this case, we must promise ourselves to do it, break out of this pattern of not showing up, and let our masculine shift into a new habit.

It is also possible that the desire to run, get fit, change our eating, or start a new habit didn't come from the feminine at all. It might have come out of our masculine intellect, and we are trying to impose it upon our feminine. Maybe we read a book or heard a speaker and got a bit high on the ideas. Our masculine then made a plan but never checked with our feminine truth. So, when morning came, half of us (the feminine) wasn't on board at all because they were never consulted and would not have agreed to it.

There's also the possibility that we simply rebel against all that is masculine. Even when our own masculine makes a plan to support our feminine truth, that rebel says, "NO! I'm not doing it!" No matter what great things we create for ourselves, we have a self-sabotage program that won't let us step forward. We refuse to connect with that masculine to help it get stronger and let us grow.

This takes us down a different path of healing where we have to unearth this blanket distrust of the masculine. The big question we must ask ourselves is: "Who are we rebelling against?"

Sometimes, we are rebelling against our parents. Perhaps they were overbearing and saw their children as extensions of themselves. If we succeed at something, we know that they would somehow take credit. This can cause us to unconsciously not allow ourselves to succeed and follow through on what our inner masculine has created for us. The key is to look at our child-self who wasn't given credit for their accomplishments and who they were with kindness and compassion. Then, we can move forward into current time and know in our hearts that all of our accomplishments are our own. We can enjoy our masculine's plan for us and start to say "Yes" to ourselves. We start with baby steps, creating that connection and trust a little bit more with each step.

I personally have spent a lot of time rebelling against the ideals of society. For my whole life, I have heard that you are supposed to be skinny, strong, and look a certain way. Therefore, there have been many times when my masculine made a great plan to get healthy through a new fitness or diet regime. What happened? Nothing. I did it for a while and then found an excuse to stop—over and over again. This repeated pattern made me look inside and ask myself why I was actually making this new plan. Was it to conform to what society thought was acceptable? Or was it for myself? Once I discarded the plans that were to look good for others and I was actually doing things for my own health, comfort, and happiness, it was a lot easier to get up in the morning and go for that run or do my yoga!

Yoga is another great example of my journey of trusting my inner masculine. I first discovered kundalini yoga through a DVD I bought online. I was instantly enraptured with this yoga! I ordered every kundalini yoga DVD I could find. I happily practiced every morning without fail. Eventually, I decided to do their teacher training program. I wanted to learn from real people and join a community. Well, I went in with my heart open and ready to learn. However, I soon learned that I didn't like the head teacher. He repeatedly told us that unless we were practising for 2.5 hours every morning, we weren't real yogis and obviously weren't dedicated to our practice. What? At this point, I had young children underfoot, cows to milk on the farm, and were often up during the night helping the cows calve. There was no way I could find two and a half hours to practise yoga and chant! Yet, every month during the training, we would be given a guilt trip if we hadn't done our "proper" practice.

Well, that was the end of my joyful morning practice. For the next ten years, I battled with my inner masculine who tried to get me to do my daily practice again. It tore me up inside that I had lost the joy or the desire to even do it. The only way I could make myself do it was to invite my yoga students to do a 40-day practice together. Because others were coming, I would make sure I was there. I wouldn't let others down — only myself.

So, it's an interesting question: "Who are we rebelling against?" To unpack this question might require journaling, chatting with friends, or finding a great counsellor. Our goal is to eventually have no one else to rebel against. Then, our inner masculine can be our amazing facilitator and cheering squad! We no longer have to spend energy rebelling against our parents, our inner masculine, or anyone else.

The Voice of Our Internal Masculine

Does your inner masculine sound like authority figures from your past? Uncaring of the real you? Critical? Judgemental?

Maybe you had overbearing parents who showed you that the masculine means aggression, anger, and meanness. We will easily internalize these experiences. The voices of our parents become the voices in our heads, and instead of our masculine protecting and supporting us, our masculine berates us and minimizes our feelings and what we desire.

Then, when we decide to do something, our masculine isn't our cheering squad. It is telling us that we had better do something, or else. This will create the same separation within us that we had with our parents or whatever authority figures we are battling.

Being aware of these voices through journaling or simple awareness allows us to start to recognize whose voices they are. We can get them to start being kinder. We can understand that those voices are meant to support our vulnerable feminine in life, not tear her down. We can find different scripts that are repeated in times of stress.

Bit by bit, our masculine will start to support our feminine, and we'll find that inner connection.

Choosing Our Role Models

Unfortunately, we seldom have great role models for the healthy masculine. In our formative years as children, we are mostly in the feminine role—child and student—and everyone else is in the masculine role. Whoever raised us, taught us, and cared for us become our primary examples for what masculine energy feels like. Sometimes, these people were wonderful, healthy masculine—protective, supportive, and strong. But more often, our parents and teachers were raised in generations of this patriarchal, domination paradigm, and that masculine energy was controlling, judgemental, and punishing.

Because of our tendency to connect the masculine with the males in our lives, our fathers become a strong example that we follow — whether we want to or not. However, it could also be a mother who was very overbearing, disconnected, and controlling. It could be a teacher, priest, or anyone who has ever been in that position of authority. They wielded the power, and were disconnected from who they were supposed to be serving. Instead, they were just separate and controlling.

When this is our experience growing up, we will often go one of two ways. We will either continue acting in the same patriarchal "masculine" way that we saw growing up, or we will decide that we will never act like that. We refuse to step into the masculine role — within or with others. We end up wanting to be neutral. We end up not wanting to do anything because it is better to do nothing than to do something that makes someone else feel bad.

So, we need to find new role models. Were there other people in our lives who were healthy masculine? (This could be anyone of any gender who embodied healthy masculine.) Were there teachers who were connected to their students and supported them in their learning experience? Were there other people in your childhood who always showed up and could be counted on to follow through?

It could even be famous people who seemed fearless. It could be Einstein who shared his theories, even though the scientific community labelled him crazy. It could be Sir Richard Branson who creates new businesses for the thrill of it, even when many of them don't make it. It could be someone who was a great father to their kids or even a political leader who had incredible integrity.

It's always interesting to read biographies and autobiographies of people our soul is drawn to. We pick up the most wonderful new patterns of who we would love to be.

Releasing the Fear of Making a Mistake

*"A person who never made a mistake
never tried anything new."*
ALBERT EINSTEIN

So why don't we step into the masculine? What stops us from taking the risk and making something happen?

We are often raised with a lot of judgement. We are told, "You are a good boy if you do the right thing, and you are a bad boy if you do the wrong thing." We want to be the good wife, the good husband, the good child, the good friend, the good person, etc. There is a lot of fear about doing the wrong thing. It is everywhere. It is the whole paradigm of good and evil.

This also comes from the belief that the only reason to do something is the end result. For example, if we start a new business, the only acceptable outcome is that it is an incredible success. But what if there is an incredibly enjoyable process in the creation of the business? What if this is a personal passion, and it is exciting to share it with the world? What if the point was to learn about opening a business? What if it was to meet new people? What if it was to hone a new part of our skillset? Obviously, we hold the hope that whatever we attempt will be a success. Optimism makes the whole venture exciting and fun. However, when we believe financial success is the only thing that is important, it can be overwhelming to the point that we get stuck and don't even try.

Other examples of stepping into something new could be putting ourselves out into the dating world, starting a new job, joining an art class, or learning a new language.

The key is to trust our feminine wisdom. When the prompting to take action comes from our inner feminine, it becomes exciting to see why we felt so called to this. We aren't attached to external benchmarks of success because our promptings came from inside, and this is a much more exciting adventure.

Social Literacy: Learning How to Read Others

Since the masculine is born out of the feminine, then we need to learn how to read others, which can often be difficult. What do they need? What do they desire? Maybe we have never even connected with anyone like that. Or maybe no one's ever connected with us like that. We have lived in a very disconnected world which makes it easy to wonder if it's even possible.

It is all about communication. If we want to help, and someone is struggling, we can say, "What can I do to help?" It is that easy to ask a question. If we're struggling in a relationship, it is okay to say, "I'd like to understand what you're feeling. How can I understand more?"

Every time we learn more about the other person, something subliminal, unconscious, and subtle happens inside. Our experience of this whole person blends into what we already perceive of them. We become better at reading people. Every time we ask more questions, every time we ask what we can do to help, we start to see signs and recognize things in other people.

Even sexually, there is the question of how you read them. We can always ask them, "What would you like right now? What would feel good for you?" When you do what they asked, you energetically connect how they are feeling with what they desired and something magical starts to weave inside of you and between you—like a dynamic reference book develops inside.

A while ago, one of my students asked me why it was so hard to read the feminine in relationships. He called it social illiteracy, which is brilliant. He told me a story that his girlfriend had told him. Her friend had gone on a date, and she thought it was going great. They were sitting on a park bench and all of a sudden, the guy just reached over, pulled her toward him, and started kissing her. She couldn't believe he did it. She didn't know what was happening. She said, "What are you doing?" He responded, "Oh, you don't want me to be masculine?"

He was trying to be masculine but wasn't reading her at all.

As my student's girlfriend was telling him this story, they happened to be sitting with a bunch of their friends. The other women chimed in, telling similar stories. He was just so shocked because he personally wasn't like that. He was more on the other side of the spectrum, struggling to be masculine because he never wanted to put anyone in an uncomfortable position.

We seem to have lost that ability to connect and read each other. We have even lost the ability to communicate, to be able to ask and find out more.

How Can We Develop Social Literacy?

There are many aspects of social literacy: what we've been taught by others, our ability to be empathic, and being clear about the ideas we have in our minds that we might be projecting onto others.

If we are lucky, our parents are our first teachers in how to read and connect with others. It could be something as simple as wanting to run towards someone in excitement but our mother senses something is wrong and puts a gentle hand on our shoulder with a look that says, "Just wait a minute". It could be learning from a friend who is "good with people" who we learn to mimic if we tend to be shy and awkward.

This learning can continue into long-term relationships where a less social person is attracted to a more social person and while easily riding their coattails in social settings, will also pick up a few tips along the way as to what feels right in the moment socially.

Empathy is the ability to sense how another person is feeling. A man in Greece once told me that he believed that humans were made of two things: mathematics and emotions. He said that it was through emotions that we truly communicate with each other. (I wish I'd had more time to talk about the mathematics part.)

Emotions are our true state. It's important to be able to feel if someone is sad, angry, happy, frightened, etc. The key is to not to think that you must change how they feel. They are just communicating their current state. This is how we read people. But because we have lived at such a distance, pretending it is a connection, how could we possibly feel these subtle nuances of another person?

Then, we must be aware of any previous baggage that we are bringing to the interaction. Maybe we're actually nervous and that nervousness blocks any ability to relax and emotionally check in with the other person. Maybe we've been hurt in the past and we have walls up blocking any real openness to the other. Perhaps we have ideas of how we want an interaction to go (like wanting the date to go well so that we end up getting sexual later) and therefore we simply project what we desire on the situation regardless of how the other person is feeling or wanting.

Developing social literacy is a huge topic encompassing our own personal healing, understanding our empathic abilities, allowing people to have their own paths without judgement, people-pleasing habits, releasing expectations, and so much more.

Being Appreciated

The appreciation of the feminine helps us to enjoy being in the masculine.

Imagine that someone does something for you. You say, "Ah, thanks. That's awesome!" This returns the energy to the giver. When we are truly appreciative, the energy pours out of us right back into them. They feel great, and more beautiful energy circulates between us.

Within a connection, everything flows and circulates. But, if you are giving and the person barely responds or notices, then the energy dies. It flows one way into a black hole. Of course, it isn't that the other person has to give you something back. This isn't an "Even-

Steven" thing—masculine meeting masculine. The feminine response is responding with genuine appreciation, allowing the energy to continue in its circuit.

If you are in a masculine position, or you have been in a lot of relationships where there was no appreciation, it takes all the joy out of giving. This can happen when you've been with a lot of "takers" in your life. The key is to find new friends, new partners, and new people... and to always ensure that you are giving something that is desired by the other person.

Becoming Rested

Sometimes we can't step into the masculine because we don't have the energy. We are exhausted—physically, emotionally, and spiritually. We just have nothing to give.

In some cultures and families, we even idolize exhaustion. People boast about how they only need four hours of sleep at night. It is the Puritan work ethic that says, "The more you work, the better person you are. You should never have to rest."

However, if you are exhausted, and you just can't give, then you can't connect either. This doesn't mean you can't be with someone. You can happily coexist and even rest together. There just won't be any magnetism between you because there's nothing in the tank to create a spark.

So, if you want the connection, fixing your fatigue is absolutely necessary. Look at your work situation. Look at your lifestyle. Communicate this with your partner and say, "I want to have a dynamic relationship with you. I want to be in a position where I'm giving in that dynamic, masculine space. I've realized that I'm exhausted. Here are the steps I'm taking to fix it. I'm going to go to a counsellor to work with them to help me deal with some of these stresses that are getting me down. I'm going to cut back on my hours at work. I'm going to make sure I go to bed on time. I'm going to cut back on my caffeine intake."

If dynamic connection is our desire, healing is important. Exhaustion is a very poor thing for us to have normalized in our society, that exhaustion is somehow a sign of success and importance. Instead, we need to be rested and clear-minded and step forward with a full tank.

Fears of Connection

One of the big reasons we struggle with connection is because, deep down, we are afraid to be totally open with another person. It's like there are always these little parts of us that we want to hold back. These are the parts of our lives that we haven't come to terms with. There's a real fear that if I am fully intimate with someone, what if that opens a window into all of me? What if they see everything—even the parts of me that I don't like?

So, we hold back. We don't give all of us. We don't lead with our whole being because we don't like our whole being, and we don't want anyone to see it. This is common. We have been taught to judge parts of ourselves. We have been taught that there are parts of ourselves that are not okay. And we have been conditioned by advertising and media that people will reject us because of those parts with subliminal messaging that says "If anyone knows this about you, you are going to be alone. So, you had better buy this product." It has been unconsciously woven into our consciousness.

So, to begin, we must ask, "Do I feel safe enough to be open with this person? Like 100%?" If the answer is "no", then maybe they are the wrong person. If they are an open, loving person, then we must look inward and ask, "What are the things I don't want them to see?"

We then learn to love those parts of ourselves—through journaling, counselling, talking to friends, or prayer. We figure that out. Because once we are wide open, it is fun to surrender to our masculine. Again, it has to be with the right person who also has that joyful, receiving spirit. If we end up doing something "wrong", we talk about it, and we roll forward together. It can't be dark and heavy. Otherwise, it is just digging deeper into those parts of ourselves we don't like.

Your Personal Journey:
1. What does your inner masculine voice sound like? Is it supportive? Judgemental? Mean? Does it sound like someone in particular?
2. Do you have fears of doing new things? Of stepping out of your comfort zone?
3. Do you have any fears of connection? Do you trust that you will speak your truth when needed? Do you fear losing yourself in the connection?
4. How easily do you read others?

CHAPTER 20

STRENGTHENING THE FEMININE

*"Feminine power isn't something we go out and acquire.
It's already within us.
It's something we become willing to experience.
Something to admit we have."*
MARIANNE WILLIAMSON

How can we strengthen our feminine side? In a world where the masculine has ruled for a long time, connecting with our feminine in a healthy way is important for all of us.

Sometimes this lack of connection shows up as boredom because we don't allow our feminine chaos. We are so over-structured and have created such comfortable lives that there is nothing unknown or mysterious left. Sometimes we work ourselves to the bone without stopping and resting or wondering why we are doing it. Many of us struggle to receive from anyone—family, friends, lovers, or the Universe.

So, what can we do to embrace the feminine and bring ourselves into balance and inner happiness?

Activating the Feminine

Someone once asked me how to activate the feminine. This is an important question because we don't actually have to. The feminine is always active. She is our creative life force. She is the life within us. We can't cultivate the feminine because she is wild by nature. She is unknown. She is mystery. She is the birthing process of everything.

The problem is that there is a cage on top of her. A big part of our journey is to understand why there is a cage and then remove it. This is why we need to redefine the masculine, not as a cage, but as a force to bring the magic of our feminine out into the world.

Being in Our Bodies

Our bodies are our feminine (all genders). They are our manifest selves. They are the vehicle that we get to play in here on Earth. Similar to other feminine dynamics, our bodies are often treated as objects. They are objects to be loved, hated, sized, compared, and improved.

Sometimes, we treat our bodies like plasticine that we can mould into something we desire—like it isn't real. We go to the gym to work it out until it looks a certain way. We don't recognize that there is wisdom in the body. We just consider it a "thing" that we are going to shape into something acceptable.

Imagine instead, that when we worked out, went for a run, or did yoga, we were listening to the body—listening to her wisdom. When I used to run a lot, I ran barefoot. One of the greatest things about running barefoot (which is one reason why a lot of people don't like it) is that you cannot force the body. You can't treat it like a machine that you are going to drive. You cannot just decide to run 5k whether your body likes it or not. You can't do that barefoot because as soon as you get tired, if you keep running, your form will falter, and you will scrape your feet.

When you run barefoot, you have to listen. You are waking up all the proprioceptors on your feet. You have to listen to what's happening in the body. You have to listen to your knees, your hips, and your back. You must be in constant communion with your body the whole time you are running.

Just imagine being in such total connection with your body all of the time. No blind forcing. Just total communion.

One of the reasons I love kundalini yoga is that it isn't competitive. Your eyes are almost always closed so you can't see the people around you. We chant, "Sat Nam," which means, "The truth within me is who I am." This mantra reminds us over and over again to listen to our truth, our bodies, and our highest wisdom. What our bodies look like in the exercises or postures isn't what is important. What is important is connecting our breath and mind with our body—as it is right now, with no judgement at all.

We need this because, we have often learned to leave our bodies. Maybe we were molested as children, and this was how we survived. Maybe it was from decades of sitting in classrooms bored out of our minds, and our imaginations were the only thing that kept us sane. Maybe it was tedious work that disconnected us from our bodies because we weren't stimulated enough. Regardless, getting back into our bodies is important.

When we are in our bodies, we can be present while making love. This is one of the great challenges for many people who want to experience tantric intimacy, but are in their heads and are not feeling what is happening in their bodies. It takes lots of practice (quite fun practice, really) to learn how to quiet the mind and fully experience the pleasure that is happening in the body.

Getting into our bodies causes us to treat them better. We are not so likely to overeat or undereat when we are connected to our bodies. We are more likely to make better food choices because we actually feel the difference it makes.

Getting into our bodies prevents us from damaging ourselves through exercise because we are not treating our bodies like plasticine to be moulded. Instead, we work with the body for long-term health and fitness, doing whatever it needs to truly thrive.

Connecting with Feelings

Trusting our feelings changes everything. Our feelings are feminine because they describe our actual reality (and we experience them in our bodies). They are the messengers who inform our masculine of which direction we should be heading and when we should be leaving a situation.

We strengthen our feminine when we practise trusting how we feel when certain things happen. How do I feel about that past experience? How we feel is our connection to Truth. If my feelings are bringing up old trauma, then it is a clue that that's where we must heal next. It mustn't be buried any longer.

This balances with a strong masculine within who holds space for us to feel the emotions without us going completely offside. Our masculine is like a good friend who listens and takes our emotional feedback seriously. Our masculine "holds space for us" so that we can tease out the truth that our emotions are showing us from any drama and confusion we may also have in our minds from ourselves or others.

This masculine creates the container for our experience so that we know that no matter how badly I'm feeling right now, I will process it, I will learn what I need to learn, and then I will come out the other side.

This brings us great peace in our core even during the depths of difficult emotional times.

The Journey from Object to Human

I've had many women come to me who were struggling with having no desire for sex with their partner. They once had great desire, but not anymore.

The challenge is that, historically, we have been treated (by others and ourselves) like objects. The human within wasn't important. There might have once been love. There might have been great sex.

But often, we were just objects playing out a role. We were seldom all of who we actually were.

One woman looking for help was very beautiful. She shared that her partner loved when she was "porn-like" and super-hot, and she enjoyed turning him on that way. For the first couple of years, she was happy to play along in their porn-like sex life. It felt good. It stroked her ego. Then, they had a child, and things began to change. She realized that she was acting. She realized that she was just playing a role that excited her husband. She was acting the wild animal part. She thought it was real because, deep down, she longed to be wild and free, but what they were doing didn't feel like that. It started to realize that it wasn't authentically her.

The true feminine is wild, and true wildness is not concerned with onlookers. Wildness doesn't play to an audience. You are simply wild like an animal. A true animal is unpredictable. You have no idea what might happen. However, when we "act" wild, we are playing out a fantasy scene where the masculine has tamed us in some way. Our wildness is focused on him for his pleasure. There is something about this that turns him on. However, he is in the total feminine energy of receiving. He has not tamed us. We are pretending to be erotic and wild with passion for him. While it may be true that we do desire sexual union, we are actually in the masculine, simply providing him with a fantasy that turns him on.

Once you see it, it feels unnatural to play out this fantasy. The fact that it is solely for our partner's pleasure becomes a total turn-off. This is the moment when you realize you are an object in his world, and once we realize that we are just an object, our desire to connect with them starts to disappear.

To shift this dynamic in our beautiful friend's case, she can still be wild and chaotic in intimacy (as we spoke about in Chapter 17) and enjoy the exploration of this freedom and pleasure. The key is for her to be authentically wild from the inside out. Her partner's role is no longer the voyeur of her "show" (even though watching his partner in total ecstasy can still be a huge part of his pleasure experience). His role is to be the strong structure that supports her flight into chaos.

In this case, she is no longer an actress (object) playing out a fantasy for him. She is her truly wild and untamed self and he is the powerful masculine who will dance with her. There are no objects here, just powerful energies playing together.

We often interact with children as objects. They are there to be moulded, set on a proper path, punished when "out of line," and made to look a certain way. This isn't a whole lot different than painting your house a certain way for the neighbours. But the child is a human. What if they have thoughts and pain and hopes separate from what you want for them? How can we want something for someone else?

If we had this experience of being treated as an object in our childhood, we need to look at whether we are still allowing ourselves to be treated as objects now, and then taking the journey within to bring our true selves out into the world.

Interestingly, we often treat good friends as whole people as opposed to objects. Sure, for some people, even friends are objects there to fulfill some purpose. But I'm talking about intimate friends, confidantes whom we trust. When we meet with them, we welcome all of who they are—happy, sad, angry, whatever. Our union is based on talking and listening, holding space when the other is vulnerable, and sometimes not being in union at all and just enjoying each other's company.

However, in marital and relationship bonds, we have a long history of a very different connection. In many cultures, the woman was an object. She was there to fill specific needs—bear children, support her husband, serve his family. She was owned and, in some cultures, totally expendable. She could easily be replaced with another who would take over her duties.

This dynamic continues to haunt us today. Many are waking up and realizing that they are simply objects in the lives of others— partners, family, and friends. But once we realize this, we start treating ourselves as real people, and dynamics change across the board.

Embracing Chaos

What would it be like to embrace chaos in our lives? We would be paying full attention to our truth, honouring our emotions, allowing ourselves to be vulnerable, being intrigued by having different ideas, and being utterly unpredictable.

Let's look at what it means to be predictable. This means that others know what you will do next and how you will react because parts of you have become robotic. They know that if they push "this" button, "this" is going to happen. If they say "that", you will react in "that" way. However, we don't want to be predictable. We don't want others to be able to control us by pushing our buttons, knowing that we fall into certain predictable patterns. We want to be alive and unpredictable! We want to be free to respond in a real way at every moment. This is being alive!

Of course, this requires us to trust chaos and the unknown. Do we fear this? Or, do we trust the infinite potentiality of the Universe? Do we trust that there are important messages within our emotions? Do we trust ourselves? This is what we truly need if we are to happily swim in the expansive chaos within.

So, we embrace our chaos within. We listen deeply and honour what we hear. Our masculine takes action based on our deep truths and our lives start to become very unique — uniquely our own. Old issues disappear because we have listened deeply to our vulnerability, and we know what we need to change. This is where the magic happens.

If you have ever seen Michelangelo's sculpture of David, it is mind-bending. It takes your breath away because he embraced chaos. He saw a single chunk of marble and just chipped away all that wasn't David. What he did doesn't make any sense. It is not reasonable. There are a million statues out there, but when you look up and see

David, every cell in your body comes alive and starts to tingle with the most incredible feeling. The hair stands up all over your body because, somehow, Michelangelo brought God down and manifested it before your eyes.

This is what happens when we embrace feminine chaos and our masculine takes action. He listens within and chips away until something our true, wild, and divine self emerges.

Deeply Listen

We access the feminine by honouring all the wisdom that our physical body, thoughts, and emotions give us. When we listen and trust ourselves, everything changes.

We are getting signs all day long. The divine feminine is always talking to us. When we slow down and listen, everything changes. We might listen to our truth and think, "Wow, this is not feeling good. I don't like the thoughts running through my mind. Something doesn't feel right about this."

We all have gut instincts that tell us when something's amok. We know when something doesn't sound right. Yet how many times do we think, "Oh, I'll just do it anyway." It's like we flip a switch inside and then ignore our truth. However, the whole time we are doing it, we have weird feelings inside like annoyance, resentment, or sadness, because we know that we are going against our instincts.

When we access our divine feminine, we empty our cup and receive divine guidance. We listen and observe the world around us. But we don't listen with our minds. We listen with our whole beings, our hearts, and our emotional bodies. We listen to the ethers and feel which way the wind is blowing.

When we receive inspiration, guidance, or ideas from this deep listening place, it is easy to have great conviction. It is easy to stand in our truth because we know it so deeply. To question it would be to question whether we had a nose. It simply is what it is. There is no question.

We can also do this with others. Imagine you are having a difficult conversation with someone. You are listening to their words and everything in between. Although the person could be yelling at you, you hear much more. You hear the words, their tone, and their anger. You hear the pain, fear, concern, and trauma. You might hear things that happened decades ago that they are reliving, and you are the current sounding board for that trauma memory. This deep listening will alter how you respond in the conversation.

If you visit a guru, intuitive, or wise woman, what do they do? They listen to your words and all the subtle impressions they get. They will feel everything in between the words you are presenting—all the things you don't want to say out loud.

We can also do this as parents in order to hear what is really going on. Maybe the kids are fighting. We could think, "Wow. They are having a bad day," or we could empty our cup and deeply listen to everything that is going on. We sit still and observe. We let other information and thoughts come in to help. We listen to the whole situation of each child to be able to understand the true nature of what's happening.

Standing in Sober Truth

> *"When the mob and the press and the whole world tell you to move.*
> *Your job is to plant yourself like a tree beside the river of truth*
> *and tell the whole world:*
> *"No, you move."*
> MARK TWAIN

If someone does something that bothers or offends you, the true feminine does not flail about emotionally. She is strong, deep, and clear. This is very important because, historically, the feminine has been framed as "overly emotional", out of control, and even "hysterical". Women's emotional responses to the patriarchal world were once even diagnosed as "hysteria" with one of the solutions was to remove women's female organs—a "hyster"ectomy—because obviously female hormones were causing her "insanity". This is still played out today with women being considered pre-menstrual, too emotional, not of sound mind, illogical, etc., which makes everything even worse and they still aren't taken seriously.

It is very important to feel whatever we feel. These feelings are our accurate response to whatever is happening. The problem is that historically, women weren't listened to. Women had no rights. In North America, women weren't considered "persons" and able to vote until the early 20th century and there are still places in the world today where women are not considered autonomous people.

Because of this, that women were often not listened to in the home (or anywhere else). So, when something was wrong in a relationship, in the home, or in the community, her thoughts weren't taken seriously. The only thing she had left was to scream and yell and act out her frustrated emotions. Perhaps this would get her noticed. Maybe this would make a difference.[4]

When we connect with our feminine, we simply know how we feel. We know that something is not okay. We know that something has to be done to make it better. As we walk forward in the world, we have to start honouring this deep feminine wisdom and just stand in it. There is no need to flail about losing our minds. We are not bound to stay in unhappy marriages any longer. We are not stuck in the ties of a clan where we will starve without them.

We are living in a different time. We have new options.

One of them is to stand firmly in our truth. If people don't like it, that's okay, because the inner feminine has no requirement to please anyone. We can move on. However, more often than not, when we simply stand in our truth, those around us will recognize

---

[4] This applies to all genders. I'm specifically referencing women here because how women have been treated historically shows us the total disregard, oppression, and misunderstanding we've had of what the feminine is.

that. They will feel the truth as well, even if it's not what they wanted. When this happens, we can have real conversations and amazing new roads are possible.

The key is to take our own feminine seriously. Trust our feelings. Connect with our wisdom. Then, stand strong in that—not in overly-emotional desperate plight. Just strength, truth, and honouring what is real.

Your Personal Journey:
1. Are you connected with your body? Do you honour *her* feelings? Do you listen when she's tired, hungry, or restless? Does she matter?
2. Do you honour your feelings? Do you believe that they are valid and important for your soul's path?
3. Have you ever felt like you were treated like an object? How about now?
4. Are you comfortable listening to your own wisdom?

A DEEPER DIVE INTO THE MASCULINE & FEMININE

Chapter 21

Removing the Domination Paradigm

"The practice of love is the most powerful antidote to the politics of domination."
BELL HOOKS

To strengthen our masculine or feminine—in relationships and within—we must notice where this domination paradigm still exists. For example, we may struggle to embrace our masculine because we don't want to overpower anyone, and we don't want to embrace our feminine because we don't want to be overpowered. Of course, it should never be the case that anyone is overpowering anyone. Yet, if this fear still lives within us, we will struggle to embrace either polarity.

It could have existed in your family. Maybe your father or mother could not be questioned. They were in charge, and that was all there was to it. Perhaps you were taught that children were meant to be seen and not heard.

Maybe it was in your schooling—you learned that other people are in charge, and you can't question them. Initially, the threat of punishment or embarrassment was enough to stop any kind of personal perspective from being shared. After a while, you stop believing that you have a say, and you may eventually forget how to access your own opinion.

It is easy to see this in the workplace. On one hand, when we are hired to do a job, it is expected that we will do that job. This isn't domination. This is simply doing the job we were hired to do. However, many workplaces are very hard to work in. Some bosses and managers are on ego trips and see their employees as being beneath them. There are managers who enjoy treating those "under them" as if they are simply chess pieces to move around.

The domination paradigm can be seen in governments all over the world. In theory, the government is there to serve the people, hence being called "public servants." But this is not the reality. Those in government are considered "in power." They often make laws to control their constituents instead of protecting them, and sometimes, they can be very heavy-handed in taking away the rights of people as opposed to serving them.

Bullying

The act of bullying is a very common example of this domination paradigm, and it is much more far-reaching than the schoolyard.

There is a lot of bullying in families at all ages. Older siblings may pick on the younger ones. Multiple siblings gang up on a single one. Bullying can be seen in parents all of the time. What are we watching when we see a parent yelling at a child? When a fully grown, six-foot-tall, 180-lb adult screams at a tiny being in their care, this is full-out intimidation. Some believe that strong-arming our children into doing things they don't want to do is considered good parenting. However, the children are simply learning how to either be controlled by others or how to bully others. Plus, they are getting accustomed to being disconnected from the parent who is forcing and bullying them. They are unconsciously learning that this disconnect is totally normal.

Beyond that, there used to be training that says we must discipline our children to do things: "Spare the rod, spoil the child." My grandfather was deaf in his right ear because, as a child, his stepfather would stand behind him while he practised piano. Every time he made a mistake, his stepfather would hit the right side of his head to correct him. I thought this was quite extreme until my daughter went on a Rotary Exchange and stayed with a family who did something similar to their children. The parents were very high-achieving doctors who wanted their children to excel in everything. So, they would stand behind their kids while they practised piano and correct them every time they made a mistake. They didn't hit them, but their kids became extremely anxious and terrified to share anything with their parents—in all aspects of life.

Bullying can also be common in marriage. It could be endless "honey-do" lists or forcing each other to go to family events. It can be guilting each other into having sex or expectations of each other that are enforced through passive-aggressiveness or true aggression.

This bullying is entrenched and interwoven into so many of our interactions that the idea of being either masculine or feminine is terrifying. We don't want to be the bully, and we don't want to be bullied. It feels much safer to just stay separate and to "stay in your own lane". But this means living in separation and this isn't what we want at all.

How to Remove the Domination

We must deeply realize that no one is above anyone else. In many ways, we are all just seven-year-olds playing in a sandbox.

We must remember that when someone believes that they are above you or thinks they know better than you, they are simply human, just like you. No matter how many schools they've attended, how many degrees they have, how old they are, or what "position" they hold in society, they are just another human playing a role. The idea that they can dominate us is pure nonsense.

We must look at whether we believe in the "royalty paradigm". Do we believe that some families are more important, or of "purer blood" than others? Do we believe that movie stars, musicians, or famous athletes are more important than "the common person"? This is an interesting pattern that might be playing in our psyches, setting us up to allow others to dominate us.

As we take this awareness into our daily lives, we start to recognize the people who want to be in that dominant position. Maybe they enjoy the power position or they believe themselves to be some kind of "royalty". We don't need to call them out for doing it. Maybe it's just their journey. The key is to simply recognize it and then realize how strange it is to place humans above other humans.

On the flip side, we must also observe if we are the ones wanting to dominate. Are we dominating our children or partners? Do we always want to have the upper hand? At home, at work, or in the family, do we always have to have the final say?

Do we like to be in the dominant position because we don't want to lose power like we have in the past? Do we withdraw and give silent treatments in order to control others? All of these are examples of how we maintain our power position.

It is the observation of both tendencies—to dominate and to be dominated—that begins the shift away from the whole paradigm. Domination only works if we believe it is reasonable. Once we look at it, we realize that it simply perpetuates separation from each other and is nothing but an empty desire for power. At that point, it's hard to take it seriously.

Learning to Trust Each Other

The feminine doesn't trust the masculine because there has been so much of this abuse and control. The masculine has used her to his advantage, benefit, and pleasure for centuries. The feminine has not been listened to or heard. Therefore, she will struggle to be vulnerable.

Many partners who prefer the masculine are not yet connected to their strength, so those in the feminine do not believe that they will rise to the challenge. Even if the feminine lets their guard down and allows the masculine energy to move, they don't believe that he will follow through. This is a huge problem.

The masculine also doesn't trust the feminine. This is part of why she was oppressed. He is afraid of being consumed by her. He is afraid of her chaos and unpredictability. He is afraid of losing his identity by merging with her.

Interestingly enough, this fear is valid. It is true that he will disappear through merging with her, but it's okay. The feminine is the physical. The masculine is what energizes the physical. It is like lightning, sunshine, or rain falling on the Earth. Lightning, sunshine, and rain are all masculine. They nurture and feed the Earth. They are important parts of the whole. But what do we see after they fall? Just the Earth. They have been absorbed. Only their effects remain.

This is the fear of serving the feminine. When we give to others, what we have given will be gone. We may not be seen in them, regardless of the nurturing effect or the benefit to the other.

This is the paradigm shift from our life's goal of building our reputation to enjoying the bliss of every moment. When we need to build our reputation, we will always be unsatisfied because there are always new people to whom we must prove our worth and impress. There is no joy in this.

However, when we just give from our hearts—meaning that we enjoyed doing it, then this is the fun. It is the thrill of being the lightning and feeling that energy coursing through us! This is what nurtures us. This is what lets us sleep soundly at night. This is what puts a smile on our faces, knowing that we have made someone happy.

Your Personal Journey:

1. Where does this domination energy still exist in your life? Are there specific places? Specific people?
2. What helps you to counter it in your relationships?
3. Do you feel this desire to dominate inside yourself? What would respect feel like instead?

A DEEPER DIVE INTO THE MASCULINE & FEMININE

4. Do you trust others easily? Partners? Family? Friends? Strangers? How does this domination paradigm fit into these relationships?

SECTION VI
Going Above & Beyond

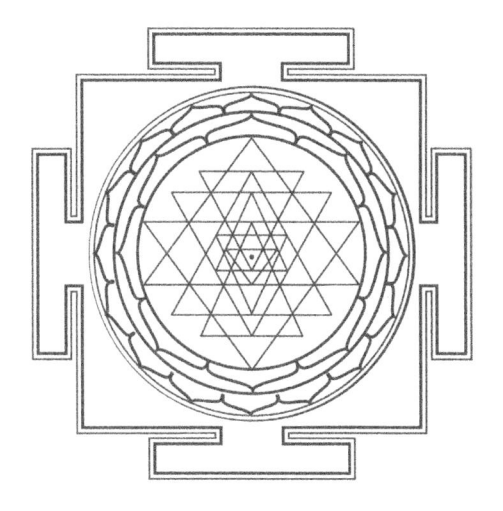

Chapter 22

An Intimate Connection with Our World

"All around you, in every moment,
The world is offering a feast for your senses.
Songs are playing,
Tasty food is on the table,
Fragrances are in the air,
Colors fill the eyes with light.
You who long for union,
Attend this banquet with loving focus.
The outer and inner worlds
Open to each other.
Oneness of vision, oneness of heart.
Right here, in the midst of it all,
Mount that elation, ascend with it,
Become identical
With the ecstatic essence
Embracing both worlds."
LORIN ROCHE, The Radiance Sutras

All of these dynamics can also be felt through connection to the world around us. This can bring a bliss state to which many of us can relate. It could be walking in the sunshine and receiving the warmth on our face. It could be watering our garden or protecting the rainforest.

Feeling union with the world allows us to feel like we are home and that we belong. Regardless of our relationship status, work, or inner health, connecting with nature is so healing and we can all do it.

Merging with Nature

There is something about walking through the woods after a rain. Wonderful smells fill your lungs. You see water dripping off of the leaves. You hear the birds singing. You feel the fresh air on your skin and the sun on your face.

Can you imagine just letting all of that in and being in full receptivity to all that nature has to offer? This is the pure bliss of union.

Similarly, we can give to nature as well. Maybe we plant trees, water our garden, and give thanks for our abundance and everything we have here. We can also protect the Earth from deforestation and pollution. There are many people who can talk to the trees and rocks. This is a real thing where they receive guidance and have full communion as if they were sitting and having coffee with good friends.

Merging with nature is like deeply connecting with our Mother. It is nestling into her bosom and trusting her completely. This is foundational for many cultures that are still connected to nature. To those who are disconnected, these beliefs don't make sense. But to those who are in union with their surroundings, nature always provides a rich and interesting conversation.

Trusting Our Divine Connection

The first time I found myself at a Quaker meeting, I thought I was going to go crazy. Most Quakers only follow what Jesus taught — that we are meant to be led by the Holy Spirit within. There are no ministers or churches. Just a gathering of people sitting quietly in a hall or someone's home, and listening for guidance.

AN INTIMATE CONNECTION WITH OUR WORLD

So, after singing some songs, everyone settled into their seats, closed their eyes, and began to listen within.

In a way, this was my first experience with meditation—complete with all of the same struggles. My mind was racing. I didn't want to sit still. How would I last a whole hour of just sitting here? I thought I might go mad.

After a while, I started to realize how much of my religious belief was strictly intellectual. I loved studying the scriptures and ideas of any religion I could find. I loved discussing faith, guidance, and what was common amongst all the beliefs. But here, I was being asked to put it into practice.

Our only goal was actual connection. This was just between me and God. No scripture. No ideas. No one else to look at how they were doing it. I had to find my way to this connection on my own.

I didn't find this easy at all. We can have all kinds of theories about connecting with the Divine, God, or Consciousness. But how do we actually do it?

We must be in our feminine. We open ourselves. We surrender. We listen. We quieten our mind so that we can hear.

When we have a true connection with the Divine, whether it is an internal Divine or an external God figure, it brings us such peace. When I am fully connected, I am able to be totally vulnerable because I understand that no matter what happens, I am not alone. I know that I'll always have guidance and inner resilience, no matter how hard things get.

One of my favourite books is Gandhi's autobiography called *The Story of My Experiments with Truth*. What I loved about this book was that he shared his inner turmoil with this very topic. On the outside, we hear about Mohandas Gandhi, the world leader who did such incredible things, but it was actually his journey of listening to God and hearing his Truth that was his greatest defining quality.

He taught about *satya*, which is Sanskrit for Truth. *Satyagraha* means to "stand in one's Truth." This is what he deeply believed and had great faith in to guide his journey. However, *satya* isn't just a personal truth at the moment. It is much deeper than that. It is the Truth that you know because it comes from Divine Guidance. There is no arguing with it because you can feel it with your whole being.

He called his autobiography *My Experiments with Truth* because he believed that if you really wanted to know him, then you should observe him when he starts to question that inner connection to Truth and God. This is where you would meet the real Gandhi.

Most of the time, he trusted his connection right through to the eleventh hour, and a miracle always occurred, but he also shared the times that he faltered and questioned everything.

When I first read this, it brought me great hope. As a perpetual seeker, I needed to hear that, even for a great spiritual leader like Gandhi, that my desire for connection with the Divine was a journey. It was a constant dance of listening, questioning, feeling deeper, taking action, and doing it all again. With each step, it gets a little bit easier to trust and feel that connection.

Eventually, it becomes the only dance we dance, and it becomes incredibly exciting and very enjoyable.

Protection & Vulnerable

Another dynamic that happens within is vulnerability with that divine, God, the Universe, consciousness, or whatever word makes sense to you. This feeling of being protected and safe affects us in all aspects of our lives.

For example, people often ask me, "How can you be so vulnerable in relationships? I don't want to be hurt. I just don't trust people."

Let's say you are in a new relationship where there's potential for real connection, but maybe neither of you have ever experienced this kind of openness before. You both want to explore it but are afraid. You sense what is possible, but you are afraid to be this open.

This is how having a deep connection within ourselves allows us to be more open and fearless with others. With a deep connection inside, we can't really be hurt. We can still feel sad and disappointed, but we also know that we will recover. This allows us to share more openly, take risks, and relax as we get closer.

Sometimes, you might be having a difficult conversation. You've realized that the reason for the issue is something quite vulnerable within yourself, and you have never shared it with anyone before. If you share it with this person, you don't know how they will react. They might be fully present, and all will be fine, but you just don't know.

Chances are it will go well. Maybe the other person will say, "Wow. That's amazing. Thanks for sharing that." Perhaps they'll be vulnerable too. Or maybe it doesn't go well. Maybe they try to use it against us or misunderstand what we say. We may go home that night feeling really hurt.

But we can pray. We can meditate. We can journal, and we can learn from it. We always get to learn from our experiences. It is not about the other person. It is always our journey. Maybe we needed to practise being vulnerable. Maybe we needed to know that we were cared for, that we were covered, that we were protected, and that we will always bounce back. This creates incredible strength inside.

Inspiration & Manifestation

This divine connection is also very practical. It is how amazing, beautiful, and new things are created in our physical world.

Let's say that we are out walking in the village, and we see a need. We observe the problem and wonder how to fix it. We ask within, and an idea comes to us. We then go out into the world and make it happen.

It is interesting to note that inspiration comes from being in the village. If we are not connected to the village, why would we ever have inspiration? Inspiration flows because it is needed. It is not about simply sitting in inspiration and meditation. It is only valuable when we are out on the earth.

Similarly, if we are having a difficult conversation, we can circle and debate endlessly, or we can ask for help within. When we do this, we will often hear guidance that is very different from what we would normally do. This, of course, is the point. As we say these new words, we get a different response from our partner. Our issue leaves the endless cycle and we both take a step forward onto new ground.

This is when we feel alive. This is when living in the world is exciting because we never know what's coming. We don't know what inspiration will come. We don't know what we are going to manifest next. It is a whole new world of possibilities.

It is also hard to be depressed when we are always inspired and manifesting. It all begins with learning how to listen, having the courage to make it happen, and truly making our mark in the world.

Pursuit & Pursued Within

The divine feminine is uncatchable. She is pure mystery, deep, and eternal. She is infinite and impossible to be grasped. Can you imagine pursuing our inner feminine for our whole life—having our inner masculine in perpetual pursuit of our deepest mystery and magic?

What a journey our own life becomes! Plumbing the depths of our desires and ideas. What new idea is rising? How do I actually feel about this situation? Is it time for change? What is arising out of the new chaos?

If the world is actually based in chaos, and all new things come from it, then this exists within us as well. This is the vehicle for all of our personal growth and journey. This is what puts a smile on our face and a twinkle in our eyes when someone asks us how we are and we respond, "I am great! I am on an eternal journey of discovering the world through my own unpredictable and uncatchable divine feminine."

Our true lifelong and exciting journey to the Self.

Exercise: Merging with God

Instead of journal questions, this is a wonderful meditation you can do. Once you experience it in this way, you can bring that feeling out into the world and feel it with the ocean, the sunshine, the forest, and anything in nature.

This exercise is one of my favourite meditations to do. It is about merging with God in full receiving, and this can result in extreme happiness, relaxation, sometimes frustration, and sometimes full-body orgasm.

The idea for this first came from a story I heard about a nun who would go to her cot every night and lie perfectly still waiting for God to come and make love to her. She knew that she had to stay perfectly still, or else it wouldn't work. When I read this, something inside of me knew it was right. I didn't know why.

During my time of celibacy, I realized that I needed to learn to receive from more than just sexual partners. So, I tried it, and true magic happened.

Now the key here is to lie on your bed perfectly comfortably. If you have pain or anything, support yourself in any way you need to relax. Your job is to relax. Every muscle, every bone, every thought, every inch of skin on your body. Just relax.

GOING ABOVE & BEYOND

Lie perfectly still. If you feel like twitching, just breathe into it. Release the tension. If your mind is rolling at a million miles an hour, just breathe deeper. Allow the thoughts to go, but don't let yourself move. Stay still like our friend the nun. Allow yourself to receive. Know that you are so worthy to receive God's energy.

Chapter 23

Becoming Something Brand New

"The whole is greater than the sum of its parts."
ARISTOTLE

We have heard this quote many times. Often, we hear it in the context of the importance of connectedness. We know that a team is stronger together. It is like there is extra mojo in the room when everyone is working harmoniously. Therefore, it makes sense to say that the whole is equal to the sum of the parts plus some extra good energy.

But this isn't what this quote really means. What Aristotle actually said was, "The whole is something <u>besides</u> the parts." This has a very different meaning.

This means that when the parts are united in a way that brings wholeness, something completely new appears. It isn't about adding the pieces together and getting more. It is about an entirely new creation from the individual pieces joining together in wholeness. The pieces, that were once separate, disappear into the totality.

For us, when we come into true union with another, we are no longer experiencing the connection of two people. We are experiencing something brand new — an indescribable love, nirvana, and joy. We are experiencing something that cannot be explained to someone who hasn't experienced it. It's special. It is totally different.

It could be sitting on the couch having a long conversation with a friend. What really happened? Was it a conversation? Were we helping each other? Or was it something else?

It could be making love in full polarity, trusting each other completely, and riding the waves of the unknown together. Eventually, it becomes unclear as to whose body parts are whose. No one knows who is giving and who is receiving. Our energies flow together until both of our bodies disappear, and we are floating through space together. What happened there? Did we make love? Did we have sex? Or was it something completely different?

We can feel this ourselves when we are deep in creative flow. I have an artist friend who creates the most incredible paintings. When the inspiration comes, she swears that the bliss she feels is greater than any kind of lovemaking. She is on cloud nine and not coming down.

Perhaps our mind can't understand it but our soul can. Our soul knows that connection is so much more important than just having someone to watch TV with. Deep down, we know that so much more is possible.

We know it is about connection. We know it is about union. We know that it is fun, exciting, and joyful.

We know that Divine Union is possible. We just need to look at the world differently, redefine the players, know that we are connected…

And get out there and play.

About the Author

Katrina Bos grew up in Toronto, studied mathematics at University of Waterloo and then moved to the country after falling in love with a dairy farmer. She was a computer programmer until babies came along and her life became about milking cows, raising children, gardening, and driving tractors.

In 1999, she went through a health crisis with lumps growing in her breast, only four years after her mom died of breast cancer. Through this journey, she met her first true spiritual teacher who guided her in a completely different way of seeing the world. This entire journey can be read in her book *What if You Could Skip the Cancer?*

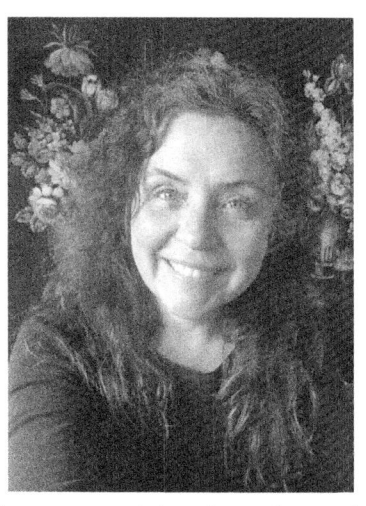

As her story spread through family and friends, people began coming to her for healing help. She returned to university to study psychology and spiritual studies. She also became a Kundalini Yoga and Meditation teacher, thus beginning a new path of counselling and teaching out in the world.

Her passion for tantra and relationships comes from her deep love of intimate connection with others—friends, children, family, lovers, students, and random people she meets on the street. This belief that so much more was possible led her to decades of study and practice of the wonderful world of Tantra and Divine Union.

Divine Union of the Masculine & Feminine is her sixth book, with more in various stages of being written. She teaches classes through her website: https://katrinabos.ca and she offers an International Yoga Teacher Training through https://satyayogaacademy.org.

You can enjoy additional teachings by Katrina on Insight Timer, an app focused on the growth for all people across the globe, where she offers spiritual talks, tantra based lectures and teachings, dance and array of human growth instruction.

Today, she lives in Goderich, Canada surrounded by her friends, children, and wonderful community. Her greatest joys continue to be the study of spirituality and humanity. She loves to dance, swim in warm oceans, do jigsaw puzzles, and take long baths.

https://katrinabos.ca
https://satyayogaacademy.org

ABOUT THE COVER ARTIST

Gina Maray is a passionate creative who loves to dive headfirst into the beauty and richness of life. Through the colors on her palette, no holds barred dance moves, loving cuddles and beyond, this multi-passionate creative is sharing her light with the world. In her paintings Gina weaves together her intention, attention, and energy with rich color to create images that bathe the viewer and their space in love and positive vibrations. Offering originals, prints, and commission art, her subjects tend toward animals and all things spiritual. Her paintings are infused with Reiki, and she often builds the energy of her pieces with layers. Symbols and words painted on the canvas are then painted over to become the final image you see.

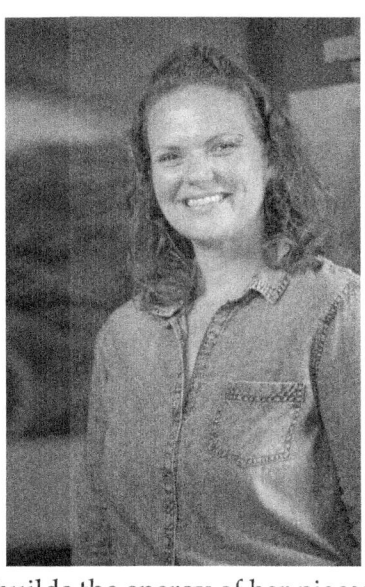

This book's cover was created in that way; you can see the process and the painting's underlayers here. https://ginamarayart.com/The-Divine-Dance_p_110.html

As a child, Gina was extremely shy and quite afraid of the world. She found solace and peaceful presence while drawing, painting, and working with clay. After earning her Bachelor's of Fine Art with an emphasis in ceramics in 2004, Gina went on to become a mother to three sweet boys. From 2007 to 2020 Gina was not creating art but was fully devoted to parenting and homeschooling. In 2020 while cleaning her basement, Gina found so many physical reminders of her childhood dream of being an artist. She heard the call of her soul reawaken, and she quickly bought some paints and canvas. Jumping fully in, Gina has been passionately painting since. The time away from art served in countless ways. It was a time of deep spiritual growth and finding her voice. Through these years, Gina has far overcome her patterns of shyness and fear.

Along with her love of art, Gina is highly passionate about Bhakti Yoga, Ecstatic Dance, Contact Improv, and Conscious Music. She loves embodiment and engaging in creative ways to come joyously into the sacred richness of the present moment. Along with being an artist and Reiki practitioner, Gina is also a professional cuddler through Cuddlist.com https://cuddlist.com/gina/. Many people are yet to realize that professional cuddling exists as a healing/therapy modality. She is proud and grateful to offer such a service that is so perfectly matched to her energy, personality, heart, and mission.

Gina is committed to living in and beaming out the energies of love, joy, play, creativity, and connection in the world, and, in so doing, helping those energies catch fire and spread.

You can follow Gina and her Energy Art here.

https://ginamarayart.com/

https://www.facebook.com/profile.php?id=100063547869542

https://www.instagram.com/ginamarayart/

Other Books by Katrina Bos

What If You Could Skip the Cancer? (2009)

Tantric Intimacy: Discover the Magic of True Connection (2017)

You Don't Have to Eat the Eyeballs: A Story of Travel, People-Pleasing & True Self-Love (2019)

Tales from the Tinderverse: A Tantrika's Journey in the World of Online Dating (2020)

Printed by Amazon Italia Logistica S.r.l.
Torrazza Piemonte (TO), Italy